ICU e-POCKET BOOK

A Ready Reference Tool for PDA Users
Version 1.0

Editors-in-Chief
Joseph Sopko, MD
Liam Alexander Briones MD, MBA,
FCCP, FAASM, FSCCM
Associate Editors
Rishi Sawhney, MD
Vesselin Dimov, MD
Authors

Liam Alexander Briones MD
Ajay Kumar, MD
Blazenka Skugor, MD
Jennifer Raroque, MD
Larisa Gamerman, MD
Loknathan Anand, MD
Lubna Salman, MD
Nabeel Sarhill, MD
Priyanka Sharma, MD
Raj Edula, MD
Roomana Akthar, MD
Shahid Randhawa, MD
Faculty Advisors
Michael Koch, MD
Adnan Tahir, MD

Disclaimer: This reference tool has been created using information from various sources. No claim is made regarding the accuracy, completeness or applicability of the information contained in this tool. This tool is in no way meant to be a substitute for your clinical judgment or other expert opinion.

1

INFECTIOUS DISEASE:
1. Biological weapons: Anthrax, Small Pox
2. SIRS
3. Sepsis
4. Pneumonia
5. CNS Infections

ONCOLOGY:
1. Oncologic Emergencies
   - Superior vena cava syndrome.
   - Spinal cord compression.
   - Hypercalcemia.
   - Tumor lysis syndrome.
2. Cauda equina syndrome

HEMATOLOGY:
1. Blood Products
2. Transfusion reactions
3. The –penias
4. The –cytosis
5. Bone Marrow Transplant
6. Solid Organ transplant

NEUROLOGY:
1. Stroke
2. Increased ICT
3. Other Neurological Emergencies
4. CNS Hemorrhage-SAH, ICH, SDH
5. Coma
6. Seizures
7. Status Epilepticus

PSYCHIATRY:
1. Suicide
2. Catatonia
3. Psychosis

CARDIOTHORACIC SURGERY:
1. Balloon Pump
2. Indications for valve replacement
3. Indications for VATS

BARIATRIC SURGERY:

MECHANICAL VENTILATION
Raj Edula, MD

INDICATIONS
From a study of 1638 pts in 8 countries
Acute respiratory failure(66%) - ARDS, Sepsis, CHF, Pneumonia........
Acute exacerbation of COPD(13%)
Coma(15%)
Neuromuscular disorders(5%)

OBJECTIVES
Improve gas exchange - Reverse hypoxia & relieve acidosis.
Relieve respiratory distress - Decrease effort & reverse respiratory muscle fatigue.
Alter pressure volume relations - Prevent & reverse atelectasis.
Improve compliance & prevent injury.
Lung & airway healing.

LUNG MECHANICS
Ppeak: Peak airway pressure: Function of inflation volume, recoil force of lungs & chest wall, airway resistance.
Pplat: Function of elastic recoil (occlude exp tubing at end inspiration).
Cstat: Compliance ie. Vt / Pplat

PATTERNS OF VENTILATION
Assist control
IMV
PCV
PSV
IRV
CPAP
PEEV

ASSIST CONTROL VENTILATION
Most widely used
Volume cycled lung inflation
Delivers set tidal volume
Triggered by patient inspiratory effort or independently if effort does not occur in selected time
I:E ratio 1:2 Diaphragmatic contractions continue & increase work of breathing

ADVERSE EFFECTS OF ACV
Over ventilation & respiratory alkalosis
Hyperinflation, auto PEEP & its complications

INTERMITTENT MANDATORY VENTILATION
Graded levels of assistance.
Volume cycled breaths at preselected rate by ventilator.
Patient can breath spontaneously between breaths.
Difficulty adapting to the intermittent nature and synchronizing with the ventilator.

DRAW BACKS OF IMV
Increased work of breathing due to high resistance from the ventilator circuit - add pressure support
Difficulty synchronizing

ACV VS IMV
Switch to IMV for -rapid breathers with alkalosis & overinflation
Switch to ACV for -patients with respiratory muscle weakness and LV dysfunction

PRESSURE SUPPORT VENTILATION
Pressure augmented breathing with set levels of pressure for every resp effort.
Allows patient to determine inflation volume & respiratory cycle duration.
 USES: Augments inflation during spontaneous breathing or overcome resistance. Popular as a non invasive mode of ventilation via mask.

PCV & IRV
PCV : Patients with neuro muscular diseases and normal lung mechanics.

IRV: PCV with prolonged inflation time
I:E ratio reversed 2:1
Helps prevent alveolar collapse but
causes auto PEEP
Used in ARDS with hypoxia or
hypercapnia

PEEP
Alveolar pressure at end expiration is above atmospheric pressure
Extrisic PEEP and auto PEEP

EXTRINSIC PEEP
Placing pressure limiting valve in expiratory limb of circuit
Prevents end expiratory alveolar collapse & recruits collapsed alveoli
Decreases intrapulmonary shunting & improves gas exchange.
Improves compliance so Fio2 can be reduced

OCCULT PEEP
Incomplete alveolar emptying during expiration.
Seen with high inflation volume &low exhalation time.
Seen in COPD & Asthma
Uses : Pulmonary oedema, mediastinal bleeding after CABG
Comlications: Decreases CO, Barotrauma
May need to use Swan ganz to monitor haemodynamics
How to detect: If extrinsic PEEP does not increase Ppeak then occult PEEP is present

COMPLICATIONS OF MECHANICAL VENTILATION
O2 toxicity
Decreased CO
Pneumonia & sepsis
Psychological problems
Dependence
Sinusitis
Laryngeal oedema
Aspiration
Tracheal necrosis
Alveolar rupture
Pnumothorax

WEANING
Raj Edula, MD

Gradual withdrawal of MV
Should be considered on every pt on MV for 24 hours or more.
Pts on MV are in the process of weaning about 40% of the time.
Spontaneous Breathing Test (SBT)

WEANING PARAMETERS

Pao2: >60mm Hg with Fio2 of 40% & PEEP <5
Vt : > 5ml/kg or > 300ml
Minute ventilation: (Vt x f) <10 li/min
PEEP: < 5cm
RSBI: (f/Vt) < 105 Maximum predictive value
NIF: More negative than -25

BASIC PRINCIPLES

Assess every pt needing > 24hrs of MV.
Perform SBT.
Minimal support during SBT(T-piece, CPAP with pressure of 5cm or less)
Consider DC if spontaneous breathing for 30-120 minutes with comfort.
Extubation is different from weaning.
Repeat SBT daily and provide non fatigable MV between SBT'S.

CRITERIA FOR SBT

Evidence of disease reversal.
Adequate oxygenation.
Acceptable acid base balance.
Haemodynamic stability.
Sufficient ventilatory drive and neuro muscular function to initiate inspiratory effort.

PROLONGED VENTILATION

Should not be considered ventilator dependent until weaning tried for 3 months.
Resources in community.
Different weaning strategies.
Slow paced with gradual lengthening of self breathing exercises.

TRACHEOSTOMY
Raj Edula, MD

INDICATIONS

Permanent neurological damage or irreversible neuromuscular disease.
Need for high levels of sedation to tolerate laryngeal intubation.
Psychological benefit
Facilitates physical therapy
>3 weeks of intubation

SEDATION & PARALYTIC AGENTS IN THE ICU
Liam A. Briones MD, MBA, FCCP, FAASM

OBJECTIVE

To understand the appropriate use and potential complications of use of sedatives and paralytic agents in the ICU.

OUTCOMES

MV →Panic, fear, agony, stress.
↑# sedation→↑LOS,↑# CTⅡfs, ↑N Pn
↑severely ill=↑sedation=↓recall
Non pharmacological anxiolysis with relaxation tapes, warm milk, herbal tea=↓need for sedation+↓delirium

ASSESSMENT TOOL: RAMSEY SCALE

Score*	Description
1	Anx, agit, restless, both
2	Coop, oriented, tranquil

3	R/. Commands
4	Brisk r/. To light glabellar tap or loud auditory stimulus
5	Sluggish r/. To #4
6	No r/. To #4

SEDATIVES
Sedative-hypnotics for sedation & to optimize a/w mgmt.
Potentiation of effects
↓BP ,cardiac fx, resp fx.
Warning: s/p cardiac arrest, hypotension, elderly, liver disease.
 Liver disease
Glucuronidation protects from liver disfx (lorazepam, oxazepam, except morphine)
Oxidation affected by ac & cr liver dz (diazepam)

WITHDRAWAL FROM SEDATIVES OR OPIATES* ≥3 Symptoms :
Restlessness
Irritability
Nausea
Cramps
Muscle aches
Dysphoria
Insomnia

WITHDRAWAL FROM SEDATIVES OR OPIATES* ≥ 3 Signs:
Myoclonus
Delirium
Sweating
Tachycardia
Vomiting
Diarrhea
HTN
Fever
Seizure
Tachypnea

WITHDRAWAL RISK FACTORS
Lorazepam 11.1mg/d
N-M blockade
Younger

WITHDRAWAL PROPHYLAXIS
Wean dose by 5-10%/d
Wean slowly if opiates and benzos used
May use long ax oral agents and wean outside the icu
 continuous infusion
Continuous infusion increases duration of ax
Rapid dev. Of tolerance to benzos

ICU SEDATION & PARALYSIS: OPIOIDS*

Drug	Lipid sol	V1/2(h)	O. Ax(')	Peak(')	Dur. Ax(h)
MoSO4	Low	2-3	5	20-30	2-7
Fentanyl	High	4-10	1-2	5-15	0.5-1
Meperidine	Mod	5-8	5	20-60	2-4
Hydromorphone	Low	2.5-3	10-15	15-30	2-4

Morphine : a-v vasodilator, histamine release, vagotonic and s-a node depresant.

Etomidate: HYPNOPTIC, NOT ANALGESIC, min effects in ventilation, min. hemodyn effects. (.2-.06mg/kg,
V1/2:3-5h, fast onset of ax)
Midazolam:
Water soluble
Antegrade amnesia
V1/2: 2.7 h, peak in 5', CNS recov 20'
.05-.2mg/kg:40%↓TV, MV no Δ
With opioids: MV also ↓
FATALITIES if cardiac dysfunction or hypovolemic!!!!

PROTEASE INHIBITORS and sedation in the ICU
Versed, and other benzos except lorazepam (ativan) and temazepam (restoril) levels are increased via inhibition of
P450 and -3A enzimes leading to higher leves of benzos. Also demerol, fentanyl, codeine and hydromorphone.

N-M BLOCKERS MECH OF AX
Depolarization of motor end plate (NMJ) by Ach→physiological conduction (very short duration)
Depolarizing relaxants (succ)→recovery over minutes→NM blockade→change in intensity of muscle response
Amplitude of depolarization decreases in a similar fashion after a dose of succinylcholine.

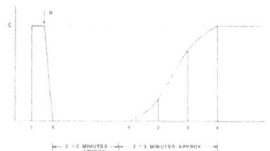

Muscle depolarization response after a dose of succinylcholine.

Non depolarizing N-M BLOCKERS MECH OF AX
Non-depolarizing relaxants (d-tubocurarine) occupy Rtors on the NMJ preventing ACH from attaching to the Rtors
sites
Change in character and intensity of muscle response

Muscle Response to the train of four test after non-depolarizing blockers. There is a change in the intensity and the
character of the muscle response.

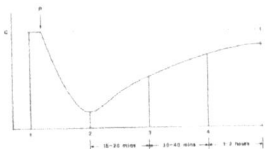

Neuromuscular blockade is prolonged after non-depolarizing agents compared to succinilcholine.

Train of four
To document that complete block is not obtained.
Four impulses are sent via two electrodes placed behind the lateral malleolus as illustrated below.

MUSCLE RELAXANTS: USES
To facilitate ETI
To facilitate mechanical vent.
To reduce ICP
To reduce WOB
Reduce spasms in tetanous

To reduce movmt in status epilepticus.

COMPLICATIOS OF M. RELAXANTS
No complications reported with use less than 2 days.
Anaphylaxis
Hyperkalemia with Succ.
Inad. Ventilation
Inad. Analgesia and sedation
Persistent weakness

Succinylcholine
Duration of ax: 5-10 min
Bradycardia
Junctional arrythmias
Ventricular arrythmias
Masseter spasm
Muscle pains

RISK FACTORS FOR ↑ K+ WITH SUCCINILCHOLINE
Burn pts.
Neurologic injury
Muscle trauma
L-t immobilization
↑ K+

RISK FACTORS FOR PROLONGED WEAKNESS WITH M. RELAXANTS
Occurs in 20% Pts on M.R for >6 days
And in 70% on pts on CST
Vecuronium in females with renal Failure
↑ dose corticosteroids
> 2 day duration of muscle relaxant administration
High dose muscle relaxants.

PROLONGED WEAKNESS WITH M. RELAXANTS
Vecuronium, pancuronium, pipecuronium (arduan): 3-desacetyl vecuronium, persists in females with renal failure.
Lt use in pts on cst develop myopathic syndrome

MYOPATHIC SYNDROME IN LONG TERM USE OF MUSCLE RELAXANTS
Flaccid paralysis
Myopathic syndrome leads to an increase in creatine kinase :. Monitor levels!
Myonecrosis
Recovery over many months

MOTOR NEUROPATHY
With vecuronium, pancuronium or atracuruim
Affects all extremities
Absent t. Reflexes
+/- muscle wasting
Moths to resolve

PERSISTENT MOTOR WEAKNESS
With pancuronium, vecuronium or metocurine (metubine)
Abnormal n-m transmission
Moths to resolve

9

TOLERANCE TO MUSCLE RELAXANTS
Can develop within 24-48 h
Upregulation of ach receptors due to chronic denervation
Minimize dosing
Give drug for a defined clinical outcome
Train-of four does not ensure that persistent weakness will not occur

PEARLS
Atracurium and cisatracurium: duration of ax not affected by liver or kidney disease
All M. relaxants may cause allergic rx, leading cause of perioperative anaphylaxis, succinilcholyne is responsible in 48% cases
Cysatracurium: Cardiovascular collapse may be the only sign of anaphylaxis

AIRWAY MANAGEMENT ISSUES
Oxygenation alone may save a pts life.
Brain damage within 3 min without oxygen
Needle in trachea for O2 until surgical a/w obtained

SHOCK
Rishi Sawhney, MD

OBJECTIVES
Define & Categorize Shock
Clinical evaluation of Shock
Vasoactive agents & Rx of Shock
Overview of Hemodynamic Monitoring
Types: Invasive Vs. Non-invasive
PA, Arterial and CV catheterization
Interpretation of Data

SHOCK
Defined as a state of multisystem end-organ hypoperfusion.

Clinical evidence:
MAP, HR, RR, Cool skin/ext., MS & Oliguria, Hypotension +/-

TYPES
Hypovolemic
Cardiogenic
Distributive
Obstructive

CLINICAL EVALUATION
Assess MAP = CO x SVR

Assess CO:
Diminished (PP, cool ext., delayed refill)
Increased (PP, warm ext., rapid cap. refill)

Hypotension + Increased CO:
Search for causes of low SVR
SIRS, Sepsis, Severe sepsis & high output states.

Hypotension + Decreased CO:
Assess Volume-
Decreased Intravascular volume
Increased Intravascular volume

CARDIOGENIC SHOCK
Low CO despite adequate venous return

LV dysfunction:
• Systolic- PTCA/CABG, volume, ionotropes, IABP.
• Diastolic- Control rate, cautious –ve chronotropics.

RV dysfunction:
• LV dysfx, ischemia, PE, ARDS, Hypoxia, Hypercapnia.
• ECHO/SG, volume, dobutamine, norepinephrine.

Valvular dysfx:
• Rx specific pathology- AS, AI, MS, MR, HOCM.

Dysrhythmias

HYPOVOLEMIC SHOCK
Decreased intravascular volume.
Loss of blood, plasma, fluid/lytes & third spacing.
At 40% loss of intravascular volume the compensatory venoconstriction fails.
Tissue hypoxia & severe injury.
Tx: Aggressive volume resuscitation, Rx underlying, correct dilutional coagulopathy.

DISTRIBUTIVE SHOCK
Normal volume, low SVR & high/low CO.
Septic, anaphylaxis, adrenal, neurogenic & vasodilator drugs.
Septic shock:
• Leading COD in nonCC ICU, 40-80% mortality.
• Tx- aggressive volume, vasoactive, ABx, EARLY ventilatory suppory, aggressive renal replacement, steroids vs. activated protein C.

OBSTRUCTIVE SHOCK
Obstruction of circulation causing low CO.
Pericardial dz, tension pneumo, abdominal tamponade, pulmonary vasculature dz.
Tx: ECHO & Rx underlying disease.
Medical Tx: volume, chrono & ionotropics.

VASOACTIVE AGENTS
No evidence regarding choice of agent.
Norepinephrine:
• $\alpha 1$, β receptors
• Preferred in septic/vasodilatory shock
• less renal injury, reliable increase in BP
• ↓ mortality compared to dopamine/epinephrine

Dobutamine:
• Powerful ionotrope, $\beta 1$ & $\beta 2$, ↑CO & ↓SVR.
• LV systolic dysfunction

Vasopressin:
• Trendy for septic & late phase h'agic shock
• Low dose (40mu/min) in septic shock.

Phenylephrine:
• Pure $\alpha 1$, veno & arter constriction, reflex ↓ HR.
• Add to dopamine, dobutamine after volume repletion.

11

Epinephrine:
- Potent ionotrope, α & β, cause mesentric ischemia

Milrinone:
- Ionotrope, potent vasodilator

Dopamine:
- D,β,α receptors, ? cause mesenteric ischemia

MONITORING
Collect'n & interpret'n of data to determine:
- Etiology of shock
- Respone of cardiopulmonary unit to therapy

Non-Invasive:
- ECHO- structural, pericardial, relating P to V
- Physical- BP, HR, Temp, JVP, Extrem, Refill

Invasive:
- PA Catheterization
- CVP monitoring
- Arterial monitoring

HEMODYNAMIC MONITORING and PA CATHETERIZATION
Rishi Sawhney, MD.

OVERVIEW
Despite use >25 yrs. & 2 million annually, no formally reviewed recommendations.
Observational studies indicated a greater mortality rate in patients with SGC.
Operator incompetence in insertion, interpretation & application of data.
KNOW WHAT U R DOING & WHY.

PA CATHETERIZATION INDICATIONS
Diagnostic
- Diagnosis of valvular disease, intracardiac shunts, cardiac tamponade, and pulmonary embolus
- Monitoring and management of complicated AMI
- Diagnosis of shock states
- Diagnosis of primary pulmonary hypertension (PPH)
- Assessing hemodynamic response to therapies
- Management of multiorgan system failure and/or severe burns
- Management of hemodynamic instability after cardiac surgery

Therapeutic - Aspiration of air emboli

CONTRAINDICATIONS
Tricuspid or pulmonary valve mechanical prosthesis
Right heart mass (thrombus and/or tumor)
Tricuspid or pulmonary valve endocarditis

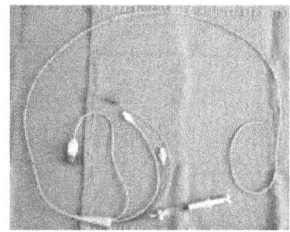

PA CATHETERIZATION: The optimal lung zone for positioning of the pulmonary catheter is lung 3 were the alveolar pressure is less than the capilary pressure and the wedge pressure represents the pressure in the left atrium. Zone 3 is reached in the dependant lung areas.

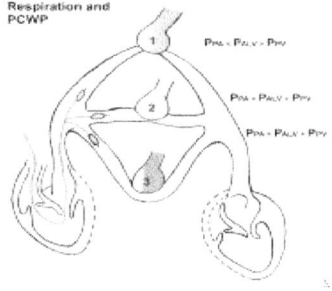

PA CATHETERIZATION: Wedge Pressure measurement.

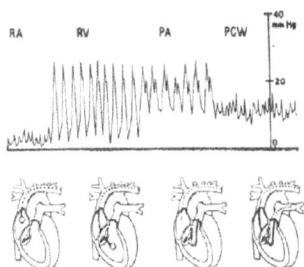

PA CATHETER: NORMAL PARAMETERS

13

Normal Hemodynamic Parameters:

- MAP - 70 110 mmHg
- SVR - 900-1200 dynes/cm square
- PVR - 80-120 dynes/cm square
- CO - 4-7 L/min
- DO2 - 700-1400 ml/O2/square meter
- VO2 - 180-280 ml/O2/square meter
- O2 extraction - 20-30%
- Qs/Qt - 3-5%
- CaO2 - 16-22 vol%
- CvO2 - 12-16 vol%

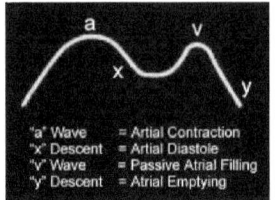

"a" Wave	= Artial Contraction
"x" Descent	= Artial Diastole
"v" Wave	= Passive Atrial Filling
"y" Descent	= Atrial Emptying

INTERPRETATION

Parameter	SAP	CVP	PAP	PCWP	CO	PVR	SVR
Hypovolemic shock	L	L	L	L	L	H	H
Cardio	L	H	H	H	L	H	H
Septic	L	L	L	L	H	L	L
Tamponade	L	H	H	H	L	N	H
RV MI	L	H	N	N	L	N	NH
PE	L	H	H	NL	L	H	H
AirObs	NL	NH	H	N	NL	H	N

COMPLICATIONS:
Initial venous access & insertion of SGC
Arrhythmias- PVC, NS VT
RBBB in 5%, preexisting LBBB puts the patient at risk for complete heart block
 PA rupture catastrophic, 50% mortality
Infection
Thrombi- pulmonary infarction

CVP MONITORING
Rishi Sawhney, MD

OVERVIEW
CVP monitoring- lower cost and morbidity
An alternative to RH Cath. in critically ill
Normal value is approx 5-10cm H_2O
Rises about 3-5cm H_2O-mechanical ventilation

14

INDICATIONS

Patients with hypotension not responding to basic clinical management ("we just don't know where we are")
Hypovolemia associated with major fluid shifts and major fluid resuscitation
Patients requring the use of inotropes

CVP Waveform

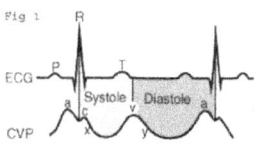

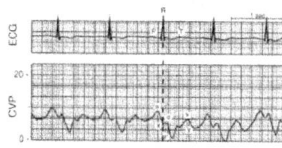

Three Peaks (a, c, v)
Two Descents (x, y)

"a" wave
Caused by atrial contraction (follows the P-wave on EKG)
End diastole
Corresponds with "atrial kick" which causes filling of the right ventricle

"c" wave
Atrial pressure decreases after the "a" wave as a result of atrial relaxation
The "c" wave is due to isovolemic right ventricular contraction; closes the tricuspid valve and causes it to bow back into the right atrium
Occurs in early systole (after the QRS on EKG)

"x" descent
Atrial pressure continues to decline due to atrial relaxation and changes in geometry caused by ventricular contraction
Mid-systolic event
"Systolic collapse in atrial pressure"

"v" wave
The last atrial pressure increase is caused by filling of the atrium with blood from the vena cava
Occurs in late systole with the tricuspid still closed
Occurs just after the T-wave on EKG

"y" descent
Decrease in atrial pressure as the tricuspid opens and blood flows from atrium to ventricle
"Diastolic collapse in atrial pressure"

THINGS TO REMEMBER
The CVP wave represents changes in pressure, not changes in volume
Mnemonic for the CVP wave
• "a" wave due to atrial contraction
• "c" wave due to tricuspid closure and ventricular contraction
• "v" wave due to venous filling of atrium

15

ATRIAL FIBRILLATION
The "a" wave disappears (no atrial contraction or "kick")
The "c" wave becomes more prominent (atrial volume is higher at beginning of systole because the atrium did not empty)

JUNCTIONAL RHYTHM
Atrial contraction occurs during systole (when the tricuspid valve is closed)
The blood has no place to go so the pressure goes up much more than usual, resulting in a large "a" wave
Cannon "a" wave
Also seen with A-V dissociation, ventricular pacing, etc.

TRICUSPID REGURGITATION
The right atrium gains volume during systole - so the "c" and "v" wave is much higher
The right atrium "sees" right ventricular pressures and the pressure curve becomes "ventricularized"

TRICUSPID STENOSIS
Problem with atrial emptying and a barrier to ventricular filling on the right side of the heart
Mean CVP is elevated
"a" wave is usually prominent as it tries to overcome the barrier to emptying
"y" descent muted as a result of decreased outflow from atrium to ventricle

Pericardial Constriction
Limited venous return to heart, elevated CVP, end-diastolic pressure equalization in all cardiac chambers
Prominent "a" and "v" waves, steep "x" and "y" descents
Characteristic M or W pattern, dip and plateau (square root sign)

Cardiac Tamponade
Changes in atrial and ventricular volumes are coupled, so total cardiac volume does not change when blood goes from atrium to ventricle
CVP becomes monophasic with a single, prominent "x" descent with a muted "y" descent
Similar to pericardial constriction but not exactly the same

ARTERIAL MONITORING
Rishi Sawhney, MD
Invasive:
Allows continuous monitoring & waves.
Repeat blood sampling.
Reliable/accurate in pts. With vasoconstriction, shock & on vasodilators.
Risk of complications- thrombosis, ischemia, embolism & necrosis.
Expensive, skilled operator & nursing.
Radial, femoral, axillary arteries

ACUTE RESPIRATORY DISTRESS SYNDROME
Shahid Randhawa, MD
DEFINITION
Acute onset of respiratory failure from acute lung injury
Bilateral infiltrates on frontal X-ray
Absence of elevated left heart filling pressures ex: PAOP < 18 mmHg
PaO_2/FIO_2 < 200 mmHg

PATHOPHYSIOLOGY
- Damage to the capillary endothelium & alveolar epithelium
- Permeability defect -> flooding of alveoli with fluid and inflammatory cells, increased inflammatory cytokines
- Collapse and/or filling of alveoli, resulting in perfusion of non ventilated airways, Blood interfaces with non functioning alveoli effecting a right to left shunt

16

- Surfactant dysfunction & reduced Lung compliance
- Decreased functional residual capacity
- Impaired gas exchange result in severe and refractory hypoxemia that is refractory to O2 therapy
- Mechanical ventilation usually required

Direct lung Injury	Indirect lung Injury
-Pneumonia	-Sepsis
-Aspiration	-Severe trauma
-Near drowning	-Multiple transfusions
-Pulmonary contusion	-Drug over dosage
-Inhalation Injury	-Acute pancreatitis
	-Cardiopulmonary bypass

CLINICAL MANIFESTATIONS
Rapid onset of severe dyspnea that lasts 12 to   48 hours
Anxiety & Labored breath
Cyanosis & tachypnea
Hypoxemia
Tachycardia
Diffuse rales in chest

PHASES
Injury or exudative phase 24 – 48 hours after injury or insult
Reparative or proliferative phase 1 – 2 weeks after initial injury
If this phase continues widespread fibrosis results
Progression Varies
Some survive acute phase and recover in a few days
Others go on to fibrotic stage with poor   survival rate

DIAGNOSTIC FINDINGS
Refractory hypoxemia
Diffuse bilateral interstitial and alveolar infiltrates
PCWP < 18
Decreased lung compliance
Assessment of Oxygenation
Pulse oxymetry
Arterial blood gas analysis
Oxyhemoglobin dissociation curve
Alveolar - arterial oxygen gradient
$PAO_2 = FIO_2(PB - PH_2O) - PaCO_2/R$
$PAO_2 - PaO_2 = A - a$ gradient
PaO_2/FIO_2

MANAGEMENT
Identify and treat underlying condition
Cultures & Antibiotics
ET & ventilator usually necessary
Low volume with PEEP should be employed
Higher airway pressures usually necessary
Give lowest possible level of O2 to prevent toxicity

INOVATIVE THERAPIES
- Prone position (enhances lower lobe recruitment & reduce VALI)
- High frequency ventilation (small tidal volume at high frequencies)

- ECMO (Allowing the lung to rest)
- Inhaled Nitric Oxide (vasodilates vessels which sub serve ventilated alveoli)

COMPLICATIONS
Infection
Pulmonary emboli
Stress ulcers
Ileus
Decrease cardiac output
Disseminated intravascular coagulation

PULMONARY SEQUELAE
A fourth of pts show no impairment
A fourth moderate impairment
Half only mild impairment
A small fraction severe impairment
Exertional dyspnea most common symp
Reduced DLco most common pulmonary function abnormality

POSITIVE AIRWAY PRESSURE
Liam A. Briones MD, MBA, FSCCM, FCCP, FAASM

PAP USES
NIVV
Splint Airway In Sleep-Disordered Breathing (SDB)
? Atelectasis

PAP IN NIVV
Works Like The Vent In Ps Mode With PEEP
S/T mode
Patients That Hypoventilate
PAP in SDB
The pharynx works as a conduit for air durign breathing and for food during deglutition
It needs to be flexible
Some people tend to collapse this conduit during sleep leading to obstruction=OSA

AIRWAY SPLINTING with CPAP

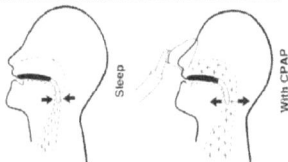

SDB RISK FACTORS
Obesity, age, male sex, post menopausal
Narrow conduit
Fam. Hx
HTN
DM
CHF, ESRD, Stroke
Other Sleep Disorders

PAP IN SDB
The goal is to provide the right amount of pressure that will keep the pharynx open during sleep.
If the patient hypoventilates, a rate will be needed.
Eliminate snoring, desat's and apneas/hypopneas.
SDB
Sleep is dynamic
The different stages may require different amounts of CPAP.
Worse snoring in s3 & 4
Worse desats during REM.

SDB COMPLICATIONS
Pulmonary HTN
Systemic HTN
Day time fatigue
Obesity
CHF
Stroke
Leg edema, and any other related to intermitent hypoxia.
Impotence, depression

AIRWAY MANAGEMENT
RAPID SEQUENCE INTUBATION (RSI)
Liam A Briones MD, MBA, FCCP, FAASM

OUTLINE
Indications of endotracheal intubation.
RSI
BV complications
Algorithms

DECISION TO INTUBATE
Is there failure of a/w maintenace or protection?
Is there a failure of ventilation (increase in pCO2, apnea, decreased RR) or Oxygenation?
What is the anticipated clinical course?

RSI DEFINITION
Simultaneous paralysis and sedation for tracheal intubation without the use of bag ventilation.
Assumes that the pt. has not fasted.
Medications are preceded by pre-oxygenation.

RSI PHASES
1. Pre-oxygenation
2. Pre-treatment
3. Paralysis and induction
4. Placement of ETT.

INDICATIONS & CONTRAINDICATIONS
Modern emergency airway management.
Difficult intubation-relative contraindication, requires to plan ahead.

TECHNIQUE
Prepare before sequence initiated
Assess airway : awake
L: look
E: Evaluate

M: Mallanpati airway classification
O: Obstruction upper a/w
N: Neck mobility

LOOK/EVALUATE THE "3-3-2 RULE"
- C-sp. Mobility
- 3 fingers between incisors
- 3 fingers between chin and hyoid bone (longer dimension, elongates oral axis, shorter dimension indicates that the larynx is tucked up under base of large tongue). This measurement will tell us if there is enough space for a normal tongue?
- Larynx in infancy is at C3,4. By age 8-9 at C5,6. Hence axix is short and the tongue will be in the way.
- 2 fingers between top of Thyroid C. and Jaw.
- Teeth: remove false teeth. Large upper incisors may obstruct, jagged teeth may lacerate the balloon.
- Oral dimension: narrow face and high arched palate. Decreased space from side to side and increased AP dimension indicates difficulty aligning oral axis.

MALLAMPATI A/W CLASSIFICATION: From I to IV.
oropharynx, pillars
IV. Soft pallate meets the tongue. II and III are in between.
Pt. must be seated, extend head, open and stick tongue out as much as possible.
Best predictor of difficult a/w.

RSI 5 P'S
Prepare
PreOxygenate
Pretreat
Place tube
Post-intubation management

RSI PRETREATMENT
L.O.A.D 3 min prior to paralysis.
Lido: Decreases ICP and A/w reactivity
Opiates: decreases ICP and preload (not in kids)
Atropine: in children only (<18 yo)
Defasciculating agents: 10% of paralyzing dose. Blocks succynilcholine induced raise in ICP

RSI HELPFUL MANEUVERS
BURP maneuver: Back, Up, R and post push by helper of patient's larynx to help visualize cords
Sellick maneuver.

UNIVERSAL AIRWAY MANAGEMENT ALGORITHM

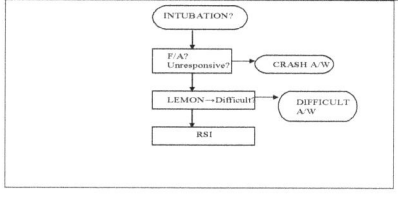

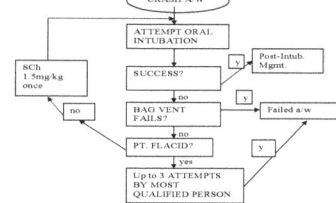

COMPLICATIONS OF BAG VENTILATION

Bag ventilation leads to gastric distention which in turn leads to aspiration.
Excesive gastric distention may lead to perforation!!!
Bagging must be done with simultaneous cricoid pressure to obliterate the esophagus and prevent gastric distention.

LIFE THREATING AIRWAY LIMITATION
AUTO PEEP
Liam A Briones MD, MBA, FCCP, FSCCM, FAASM

CONCEPTS

- Airway obstruction +/- inflammation &/or loss of elastic recoil leads to expiratory airflow limitation & air trapping.
- This leads to increase in lung volume which in turn distends the airways.
- At the same time this leads to the generation of high alveolar pressure which sometimes exceeds atm. pressure at end exhalation generating intrinsic PEEP(Auto PEEP):Elevation of alveolar pressure above Atm. P. at end exhalation.
- This might exist at resting states in patients with airway obst.,but it increases during acute attacks(2ry to inf.,drugs,allergens…),or if exhalation time is shortened.
- Airway obst. Can also be caused by narrow or kinked ETT,secretions or agitation.
- All that increases the WOB and leads to ventilatory failure.
- That also increases intrathoracic pressure and decreases the venous return.
- Auto PEEP is ideally measured on sedated patients by occluding the mouth piece at end exp. And measuring the pressure at the mouth end=Alv.pressure.

TREATING AUTO PEEP

In spontaneous breathing: Ask the patient to exhale slowly.
In ventilated patients: CPAP or PEEP,decrease resp. rate,decrease TV. This will decrease the WOB. Which will decrease CO2 production.

AMOUNT OF PEEP

Should be less than the Auto PEEP,and usually that is <15 cm H2O.
Higher PEEP will cause patient discomfort and anxiety 2ry to lung over expansion.
Auto PEEP is dynamic so PEEP should be adjusted during the course of the illness.

21

CONTRAINDICATIONS
Unilateral lung disease.
Elevated peak and mean airway pressures.
Bronchopleural fistula.
Hypovolemia.
Raised ICP.
6-P.E.

VENTILATIORY THERAPY
- Invasive.
- NIPPV.
- Hypoxemia during COPD/Asthma exacerbation results from decreased alv. vent. and V/Q mismatch. Accordingly small increases in alv. oxygen tension markedly improves PaO2.(use least amount of O2).

DRUG THERAPY
1-Bronchodilators:
-Inhaled B2 agonists_ MDI is preferred.
given Q 2-4 hours.
no S/Q or oral use.
-Inhaled anticholinergics:
Q 4hours(last longer).
2-Systemic corticosteroids:
0.5 mg/Kg I.V. Q 6 hours.
can be stopped abruptly if used for 72 hours,unless the patient was on chronic steroids.
3-Inhaled steroids:
less effective,used for stable patients.
4-Antibiotics:
Against H.flu.Pneumococci and M.cataralis.
5-Core pulmonale Rx.
6-Theophylline,mucolytics,S/Q or I.V. B2 agonists are not indicated.

ABG PATHWAY
Liam ABriones MD, MBA, FCCP, FAASM
POST INTUBATION
1. Vent settings:
- TV 5cc/kg (ideal body weight) _____
- RR =10 (liters/min)/TV
- FIO2=100%

2. POX + end-Tidal CO2 30 ' later, keep POX>94%, ETCO2
3. Sedation
4. Insert NGT + start feedings right away unless contraindicated!!!
5. Foley to gravity
6. Pepcid (if fails, Protonix)
7. Continuous Pox monitoring.

INDIRECT CALORIMETRY
Liam A Briones MD, MBA, FCCP, FAASM
OBJECTIVES
- To raise awareness of the importance of proper nutrition in the ICU.
- To understand the clinical applications of indirect calorimetry.
- To apply the results in the clinical setting.

BACKGROUND
- Protein-calorie malnutrition is prevalent in hospitalized patients. (Iatrogenic!)

22

- Hormonal adaptation follows inadequate intake.
- 70Kg man: 30K Kcal from muscle and 1200 Kcal from Glycogen stores.
- Further depletion if critically ill.
- Protein-calorie malnutrition alters normal lung function.
- The end result is that the normal lung functionally becomes diseased lung.
- COPDers are malnourished already, critical illness amplifies pulmonary dysfunction.
- Proper Nutrition is critical.

EFFECTS OF CLINICAL STRESS ON TEE

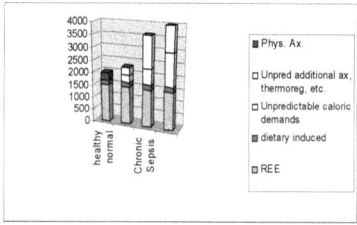

Healthy normal, major surgery, chronic sepsis and thermal Injury effects on Total Energy Expenditure.

Effects of improper diet
Excess calories in general, and excess CHO's in particular, act as metabolic stress.
O2 Consump. And CO2 prod increases.
Increases demand in lung function
MEETING requirements is essential.

DEFINITIONS
- VO2= SV x HR x a-vO2 diff=300 ml/' rest.
- Calorie: unit of heat production. It is a measure of work and energy.
- Calorie: measure of power of rate of energy utilization. 1 cal= 200 ml of O2 consumption, 1 lit O2 cons produces 5 calories.
- RER=respiratory exchange ratio when measured for the entire organism and it is know as the respiratory quotient (RQ) when measured at the cellular level.

CLINICAL APLICATION
- IC decreases the variability and prediction errors of estimation methods (Harris-Benedict equation) in determining the nutritional requirements in these pts.
- RER=Vol CO2 produced/Vol O2 consum.
- CHO= RER=6CO2/6O2=1
- Fat=RER=0.70
- Prot=RER=0.80

RER physiologic range= .70-1.0
RER>.85: give more lipids
RER <0.85: give more CHO.

NUTRITION IN THE ICU
Ajay Kumar, MD
BENEFITS OF NUTRITIONAL SUPPORT
Preservation of nutritional status
Prevention of complications of protein malnutrition
Post-operative complications

23

WHO REQUIRES NUTRITIONAL SUPPORT?
Patients already with malnutrition - surgery/trauma/sepsis
Patients at risk of malnutrition

PATIENTS AT RISK OF MALNUTRITION
Depleted reserves
Cannot eat for > 5 days
Impaired bowel function
Critical Illness
Need for prolonged bowel rest

NUTRITIONAL ASSESSMENT: HOW DO WE DETECT MALNUTRITION?
History
Physical examination
Anthropometric measurements
Laboratory investigations

NUTRITIONAL ASSESSMENT:HISTORY
Dietary history
Significant weight loss within last 6 months
> 15% loss of body weight
compare with ideal weight
Beware the patient with ascites/ oedema

TYPES OF NUTRITIONAL SUPPORT
Enteral Nutrition
Parenteral Nutrition

ENTERAL FEEDING IS BEST
More physiologic
Less complications
Gut mucosa preserved
No bacterial translocation
Cheaper

ENTERAL FEEDING IS INDICATED
When nutritional suport is needed
Functioning gut present
No contra-indications
no ileus, no recent anastomosis, no fistula

TYPES OF FEEDING TUBES
Naso-gastric tubes
Oro-gastric tubes
Naso-duodenal tubes
Naso-jejunal tubes

TYPES OF FEEDING TUBES
Gastrostomy tubes
    Percutaneous Endoscopic Gastrostomy (PEG)
    Open Gastrostomy
Jejunostomy tubes

WHAT CAN WE GIVE IN TUBE FEEDING?
- Blended foods
- Commercially prepared feeds

- Polymeric eg. Isocal, Ensure, Jevity
- Monomeric / elemental eg Vivonex

COMPLICATIONS OF ENTERAL FEEDING
12% overall complication rate
- Gastrointestinal complications
  - Distension
  - Nausea and vomiting
  - Diarrhoea
  - Constipation
  - Intestinal ischaemia
- Infectious
  - Aspiration Pneumonia
  - Bacterial contamination
- Mechanical
  - Malposition of feeding tube
  - Sinusitis
  - Ulcerations / erosions
  - Blockage of tubes
- Metabolic

PARENTERAL NUTRITION
Allows greater caloric intake
BUT
Is more expensive
Has more complications
Needs more technical expertise

WHO WILL BENEFIT FROM PARENTERAL NUTRITION?
Patients with abnormal gut function
Cannot consume adequate amounts of nutrients by enteral feeding
Are anticipated to not be abe to eat orally by 5 days
Prognosis warrants aggressive nutritional support

TWO MAIN FORMS OF PARENTERAL NUTRITION
Peripheral Parenteral Nutrition
Central (Total) Parenteral Nutrition

PERIPHERAL PARENTERAL NUTRITION
Given through peripheral vein
short term use
mildly stressed patients
low caloric requirements
needs large amounts of fluid
contraindications to central TPN

WHAT TO DO BEFORE STARTING TPN
Nutritional Assessment
Venous access evaluation
Baseline weight
Baseline lab investigations

VENOUS ACCESS FOR TPN
Need venous access to a "large" central line with fast flow to avoid thrombophlebitis

BASELINE LAB INVESTIGATIONS
Full blood count
Coagulation screen
Screening Panel # 1
Ca^{++}, Mg^{++}, PO_4^{2-}
Lipid Panel # 1
Other tests when indicated

STEPS TO ORDERING TPN
1. HOW MUCH VOLUME TO GIVE?
- Cater for maintenance & on going losses
- Normal maintenance requirements
- By body weight
- alternatively, 30 to 50 ml/kg/day
- Add on going losses based on I/O chart
- Consider insensible fluid losses also
- eg add 10% for every ^{o}C rise in temperature

2. CALORIC REQUIREMENTS
BASED ON TOTAL ENERGY EXPENDITURE
- Can be estimated using predictive equations
TEE = REE + Stress Factor + Activity Factor
- Can be measured using metabolic cart

Caloric requirements
Stress Factor
Caloric requirements
Activity Factor
Caloric requirements
REE Predictive equations

Harris-Benedict Equation
Males: REE = 66 + (13.7W) + (5H) - 6.8A
Females: REE= 655 + (9.6W) + 1.8H - 4.7A

Schofield Equation
25 to 30 kcal/kg/day

HOW MUCH CHO & FATS?
- "Too much of a good thing causes problems"
- Not more than 4 mg / kg / min Dextrose
(less than 6 g / kg / day)
Rosmarin et al, Nutr Clin Pract 1996,11:151-6
- CHO usually form 70-75 % of calories

HOW MUCH FATS?
- Not more than 0.7 mg / kg / min Lipid
(less than 1 g / kg / day)
Moore & Cerra, 1991
- Fats usually form 25 to 30% of calories

- Not more than 40 to 50%
- Increase usually in severe stress
- Aim for serum TG levels < 350 mg/dl or 3.95 mmol / 1

HOW MUCH PROTEIN TO GIVE?
Based on calorie : nitrogen ratio
Based on degree of stress & body weight
Based on Nitrogen Balance

CALORIE : NITROGEN RATIO
Normal ratio is
150 cal : 1g Nitrogen

Critically ill patients
85 to 100 cal : 1 g Nitrogen in

Based on Stress & BW
- Non-stress patients   0.8 g / kg / day
- Mild stress   1.0 to 1.2 g / kg / day
- Moderate stress 1.3 to 1.75 g / kg / day
- Severe stress   2 to 2.5 g / kg / day

Based on Nitrogen Balance
Aim for positive balance of
1.5 to 2g / kg / day

Electrolyte Requirements
Cater for maintenance + replacement needs

Na^+	1 to 2 mmol/kg/d	(or 60-120 meq/d)
K^+	0.5 to 1 mmol/kg/d	(or 30 - 60 meq/d)
Mg^{++}	0.35 to 0.45 meq/kg/d	(or 10 to 20 meq /d)
Ca^{++}	0.2 to 0.3 meq/kg/d	(or 10 to 15 meq/d)
PO_4^{2-}	20 to 30 mmol/d	

TRACE ELEMENTS
Total requirements not well established
Commercial preparations exist to provide RDA
- Zn   2-4 mg/day
- Cr   10-15 ug/day
- Cu   0.3 to 0.5 mg/day
- Mn   0.4 to 0.8 mg/day

OTHER ADDITIVES
- Vitamins
- Give 2-3x that recommended for oral intake
- us give 1 ampoule MultiVit per bag of TPN
- MultiVit does not include Vit K
- can give 1 mg/day or 5-10 mg/wk

OTHER ADDITIVES

- Medications
- Insulin
    - can give initial SQ Insulin based on sliding scale according to acucheck q6h (keep <11 mmol/l)
    - once stable, give 2/3 total requirements in TPN & review daily
    - alternate regimes
        – 0.1 u per g dextrose in TPN
        – 10 u per liter TPN initial dose
- Other medications

TPN MONITORING
Clinical Review
Lab investigations
Adjust TPN order accordingly

CLINICAL EVALUATION:
clinical examination
vital signs
fluid balance
catheter care
sepsis review
blood sugar profile
Body weight

LAB INVESTIGATIONS:
Full Blood Count- weekly, unless indicated
Renal Panel # 1- daily until stable, then 2x/wk
Ca^{++}, Mg^{++}, PO_4^{2-} - daily until stable, then 2x/wk
Liver Function Test- weekly
Iron Panel- weekly
Lipid Panel- 1-2x/wk
Nitrogen Balance- weekly

NUTRITIONAL BALANCE
Nutritional Balance = N_{input} - N_{output}
1 g N   = 6.25 g protein
N_{input} = (protein in g ⌐ 6.25)
N_{output} = 24h urinary urea nitrogen + non-urinary N losses
            (estimated normal non-urinary Nitrogen losses about 3-4g/d)

COMPLICATIONS RELATED TO TPN
Mechanical Complications
Metabolic Complications
Infectious Complications

MECHANICAL COMPLICATIONS
pneumothorax
air embolism
arterial injury
bleeding
brachial plexus injury
catheter malplacement
catheter embolism
thoracic duct injury

METABOLIC COMPLICATIONS

Abnormalities related to excessive or
inadequate administration
hyper / hypoglycaemia
electrolyte abnormalities
acid-base disorders
hyperlipidaemia

METABOLIC COMPLICATIONS
Hepatic complications
Biochemical abnormalities
Cholestatic jaundice
•too many calories (carbohydrate intake)
•too much fat
Acalculous cholecystitis

INFECTIOUS COMPLICATIONS
Insertion site contamination
Catheter contamination
improper insertion technique
use of catheter for non-feeding purposes
contaminated TPN solution
contaminated tubing
Secondary contamination – septicaemia

STOPPING TPN
Stop TPN when enteral feeding can restart
Wean slowly to avoid hypoglycaemia
Monitor hypocounts during wean
Give IV Dextrose 10% solution at previous infusion rate for at least 4 to 6h
Alternatively, wean TPN while introducing enteral feeding and stop when enteral intake meets TEE

ACID-BASE ANALYSIS
Nabeel Sarhill, MD

- **STEP 1**
  - Determine whether pt is acidemic or alkalemic, (ph 7.35-7.45)
- **STEP 2**
  - Is acid-base disturbance due to primary resp* or meta disorder {Pa co2 (35-45), HCO3 (24+2 meq/dl)}
- **STEP 3** if resp disturbance? Chronic or acute!!
- **STEP 4** if meta acidosis? AG or non-AG!!
- **STEP 5** if meta disturbance? Resp compensation!!
- **STEP 6** if ag meta acidosis? Any other metabolic disturbance!!

TYPES OF ACIDOSIS/ALKALOSIS

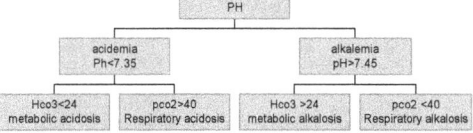

29

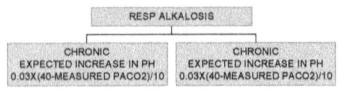

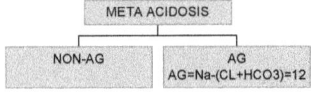

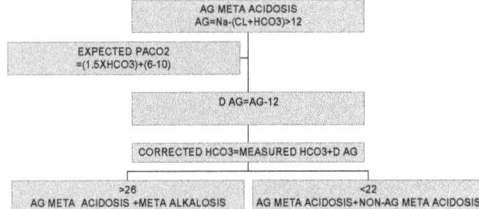

HYPERBARIC OXYGEN THERAPY
Blazenka Skugor,MD

PRINCIPLE
- Henry's Law states that amount of gas dissolved in solution is directly proportional to its partial pressure.
- Oxygen carrying capacity of blood depends mainly on hemoglobin, however O2 itself can dissolve in blood
- At 1Atm(760mmHg) 1.5mL of O2 is dissolved in mL/blood
- At 3Atm 6mL of O2 per mL of blood is dissolved
- Interaction of Hyperbaric oxygen with carboxyhemoglobin (COHb)
- Half life of COHb in room air is 4-5 hours
- Half life of COHb in 100% oxygen is 80 minutes
- At 2.5Atm hyperbaric oxygen the half life of COHb is reduced to less then 25 minutes
- Reduces half life of CO cytochrome c oxydase complex
- Inhibits release of toxic metabolits from neutrophils
- Side effects, generally minimal for treatments <120 min at 3Atm

INDICATIONS
CO poisoning
Decompression sickness and air embolism
Gas gangrene, necrotizing fascitis
Nonhealing wounds, compromised skin flaps
Radiation injury
Crush injuries,compartment syndromes

COMPLICATIONS
Reversible myopia
Middle ear effusions
Pulmonary barotrauma

Pulmonary oxygen toxicity
Seizures

CO POISONING, INDICATIONS FOR THERAPY
COHb>20-40%
Any symptomatic CO poisoning
Loss of consciousness, neurological signs
Pregnant women Hb-CO>20% (controversial - published experience is limited)
History of CAD and Hb-CO level>20%
Leading cause of death by poisoning in USA(5-6000 per year)

PROPERTIES OF CO
CO odorless, tasteless, colorless gas
With hemoglobin – carboxyhemoglobin (COHb) non-smokers <3%, smokers 2.5-10%
Affinity >240 x of oxygen for hemoglobin
Half life: RA 240 min, 100% oxygen 80 min 3 Atm 20-30 min

METABOLISM OF CO
Inhaled CO-absorbed and eliminated trough lungs
Less then 1% is oxidized to carbon dioxide
10-15% is bound to proteins

CO TOXICITY
Alteration of dissociation characteristics of oxyhemoglobin (shifts to left), binding of CO
        to Hb will increase its affinity for oxygen
Direct CO toxicity to tissues
Decreased cellular O^2 utilization – binds to cytochrome c oxidase and cytochrome P-450
Binds to myoglobin – myocardial and skeletal muscle dysfunction

SOURCES of carbon monoxide
Smoke from fire
Paint remover containing methylene chloride metabolized to CO by liver
Furnaces
Gasoline powered engines
Tobacco smoke

CLINICAL PRESENTATION
chronic or occult Difficult to dg
Acute Suggestive history
- Clinical effects correlate poorly with COHb levels
- Nonspecific, "flu" symptoms, headache, nausea
- CNS: altered cognition, seizures, coma delayed neuropsychiatric syndrome
- Cardiopulmonary: dyspnea, angina, dysrhytmias, myocardial ischemia
- Cherry red skin and lips (rare)
- Asymptomatic, levels less then 10%
- Mild, carboxyhemoglobin level 11-20%
- Moderate COHb 21-30%
- Moderately severe COHb 31-40%
- Severe (neurologic abnormalities – seizures)
- Extreme, COHb more then 50%
- COHb levels may not correlate with the clinical status
- Asymptomatic, levels less then 10%
- Mild, carboxyhemoglobin level 11-20%
- Moderate COHb 21-30%
- Moderately severe COHb 31-40%

- Severe (neurologic abnormalities – seizures)
- Extreme, COHb more then 50%
- COHb levels may not correlate with the clinical status

COMPLICATIONS (MORE FREQUENT)
Pregnancy – fetal Hb has higher affinity for CO than adult
Elderly pt, CAD, anemia, pulmonary disease

DIAGNOSIS
By history
Physical exam
Elevated carboxyhemoglobin measured by cooximetry (blood gas sample)
ABGs (respiratory alkalosis with metabolic acidosis)
Toxicology screen
EKG, CT head, MRI, SPECT scanning
Neuropsychological testing

TREATMENT
Administration of high flow oxygen (100%)
Hyperbaric oxygen therapy
Supportive treatment – acidosis, cerebral edema.
COHb levels are not predictive of delayed neurological sequelae

DECREASES THE INCIDENCE AND SEVERITY OF   DELAYED NEUROCOGNITIVE DEFICITS / CO POISONING
- Randomized clinical trial in Australia (191pt) no benefit from HBO, Med J Aust 1999.
- NEJM,October 2002, double blind, randomized trial (Hyperbaric Oxygen for Acute Carbon Monoxide Poisoning). Cognitive sequelae at six weeks were less frequent in the hyperbaric oxygen group then in the normobaric oxygen group.

ACUTE CORONARY SYNDROME
Discuss hx. of CAD and plaque formation
- A. Athersclerosis is 90% of cases and a chronic process
- B. Thrombus formation is an acute process
- C. Coronary spasms-drug abuse

Differentiate MI's and angina
- A. Unstable vs. Stable angina
- B. Non q-wave MI-portion of myocardium
  Not all the way through the heart
- C. Q-wave MI-involves the entire myocardium also
       called a transmural infarct

Anatomy of the heart and sx's pt. Will have
- A. RCA
- B. LAD
- C. Circumflex
- D. Left main
- E. Collateral circulation

Ischemia-inverted T-wave and hypoxic tissue
Injury-ST elevation-prolonged hypoxia
Review of how to measure for st segment elevation. 2 mm or greater is significant
Infarct-Q wave is present forever

Want to explain that the greater degree of st segment changes the more leads invorved correlates with the amount of tissue at risk.

12 lead ekg correlation with salli goes around'
Draw the picture and explain start at base of heart and go around

Go to acute coronary syndrome acute ischemic chest
Pain algarhythm and go through each treatment plan.
- Assessment-old chart mneumonic
- Mona-mso, ntg, aspirin, oxygen
- 12 lead and know what algarhythm to follow depending on if changes or not
- Drug therapy
    Beta blockers, fibrolytics, (warnings and contraindications), ace inhibitors, heparin
- Treatment options-ptca, cabg, caths, stress tests
- Enzyme interpretation-
- Cell membrane becomes permeable when injured and that is how we measure for troponin and cpk

TROPONIN LEVELS
1.5 positive for MI
Troponin levels will be abnormal 4-8 hrs. After onset of chest pain
Peak 12-16 hrs
Remain elevated for 5-9 days post infarct

CPK-MB LEVELS
Abnormal 4-6 hrs. After MI
Peak 18-24 hrs
Return to normal within 3-4 day

BRADYCARDIA
Refer to algorithm
Stress not to treat if pt. Is asymptomatic
Stress use of transcutaneous pacing early on
Use scenario in book or binder

ASYSTOLE
Stress new changes are having family present during resuscitative efforts
Want to clarify up front dnr and code issues so can preserve quality of life and go by pt. Wishes
Push for dnr if this is what pt. Wanted
If no response to resusitative efforts aha recommends ceasing efforts after 20 mins.
Confirm asystole in 2 leads and also increase size and gain to see if any activity
Jcah tracking true success of asystole even after a resusitation. Most cases pt. Will arrest again and the outcome is still the same.
Asystole-mneumonic

Have a cup of tea
T—transcutaneous pacing
E----epinephrine
A----atropine

Do a scenario and if able want to always focus on secondary causes and this can help determine extent of agressiveness with resusitative efforts

Go over zoll lifepak /go over patches and application
Defibrillation 120j, 150j, 200j/cardiovert 25j, 50j, etc.

AORTIC DISSECTION
Blazenka Sugor,MD

ANEURYSM
Dilatation of artery to a diameter at least 50% more then normal

TYPES:
* dissecting – break in in the vessel wall through muscle layer
* Saccular – usually at vessel bifurcation
* Fusiform
* Berry – in the CNS
* Familial – polycystic kidney disease, Osler Weber Rendu Syndrome

TYPES:
* Aquired – history of hypertension and high cholesterol
* Chest trauma
* Infections or inflammatory
* Inflammatory – Takayasu and Giant Cell Arteritis
* Syphilis
* Polychondritis
* Reiter Sy, Ankylosing Spondylitis, RA, SLE
* Abnormal collagen - Marfan

Thoracic
Abdominal

THORACIC AORTIC ANEURYSM
Ascending or Type A
about 60% of aortic dissections occur here
danger of dissection into coronary artery outflow tracts
Marfan's Sy is a predisposing factor

Descending
usually correctable
complication is injury to spinal artery

SYMPTOMS AND SIGNS OF DISSECTION
Asymptomatic
Wide mediastinum on CXR
Suden, knife like substernal CP radiating to back
Diaphoresis
Tachycardia, hypertension
Unequal radial pulses
SVC compression sy- hoarseness, stridor, edema dyspnea
Syncope, focal neurologic defects

DIAGNOSIS OF THORACIC AORTIC DISSECTION
Angiogram (sensitivity 90%,specificity 95%)
CT scans
MRI if hemodynamically stable pt
Transesophageal echocardiography
CXR

TREATMENT OF DISSECTION
In hospital mortality 30% (type A higher risk)
Type A need immediate replacement – high risk fatal rupture

34

ß blockers can stabilize type B dissections
Endoluminal stent-graft plecement

Risk of rupture after 5 years:
   aneurysms <4cm is 0%
          4-6cm is 16%
          >6cm is 31%

ABDOMINAL AORTIC ANEURYSM
Risk factors: age-most pt are more then 60 y old
   smoking
   hypercholesterolemia
   hypertension
   male sex (75-80%)

Risk of dissection or perforation: size >5.5cm
   surgery considered when size >5.5cm or expansion >1cm/year
   Recommend surveillance every 3-6 months until size reaches 5.5cm

TREATMENT
Acute dissection is surgical emergency
Medical therapy: ß blockers and nitrates(IV nitroglycerin or nitroprusside)
Endovascular stents
Prophylactic surgical correction

HYPERTENSIVE EMERGENCIES
Priyanka Sharma, MD

HTN URGENCIES
systolic BP >220 mmHg
DBP >125mmHg
persistence of readings after a period of observation
optic disc edema
progressive target organ complications
severe peri operative hypertension
parenteral therapy not usually required

HYPERTENSIVE EMERGENCY
DBP >130 mmHg
includes malignant HTN, HTN encephalopathy, HTN nephropathy, ICH, aortic dissection, pre eclampsia, eclampsia, pulmonary edema, unstable angina or MI.
renal failure will ensue if untreated.
prognosis same with papilledema/retinal hemorrhage or exudate.

GOALS OF THERAPY
Initial aim is to lower DBP to 100-105 mmhg over 2 to 6 hrs
Maximum initial fall in BP not exceeding 25% of presenting value
Once controlled, switch to oral therapy with DBP gradually reduced to 85-90mmhg over 2 to 3 months

IV DRUGS	DRUG	DOSE	ONSET	PEAK EFFECT	DURATION
	Nitroprusside	0.3-10mcg/kg/min	Immediate	1-2 min	1-3 min
		20mg, then 20-80 mg every 10 min	3-5 min	10-20 min	3-6 hrs
	Nitroglycerine	5-300 mcg/min	1-2 min	1-2 min	1-3 min
	Nicardipine	5-15 mg/hr	1-3 min	5-20 min (dose dependent)	15-40 min
		3-5 mg/hr			

35

ORAL DRUGS

DRUG	DOSE	ONSET	PEAK	DURATION
Nifedipine	10 mg	5-15 min	15-30 min	3-5 hr
Clonidine	0.1-0.2 mg, then every 1 hr (max 0.8 mg)	30-60 min	2-4 hr	3-8 hr
Captopril	6.25-25 mg	15 min (oral) 5 min (SL)	60-90 min 10-15 min	4-6 hr 2-3 hr

NITROPRUSSIDE SODIUM
Drug of choice
Rapid and controlled action
Continuous monitoring (especially invasive bp monitoring)
Aortic dissection (with beta blocker)
Not preffered in mi
Cyanide toxicity possible

NITROGLYCERIN
Less potent
With acute ischemic syndromes
Tolerance

LABETALOL
Preferred in pregnancy
Avoid in CHF and asthma

ESMOLOL
Rapid acting beta blocker
Approved only for svts
Less potent
Reserved for patients with concerns about aes to beta blockers
Avoid in CHF and asthma

NICARDIPINE
most potent
long acting of IV CCBs
precipitates reflex tachycardia (use with beta blocker in IHD)
can precipitate MI

FENOLDOPAM
peripheral DA1 receptor agonist
No evidence of tolerance, rebound, withdrawl or decreased renal function
Tachycardia with high dose
Increased intraocular pressure

ENALPRILAT
Onset in 15 minutes
Peak in 6 hrs
Used as adjunct with diuretics

DIAZOXIDE
Directly acting vaso dilator
No effect on renal bld flow
Given in small bolus or infusion
Use in pre eclampsia and eclampsia
Causes hyperglycemia and sodium and water retention (use with loop diuretic)

HYDRALAZINE
Less predictable
Reflex tachycardia (do not give without beta blocker)
In pregnancy and children
Avoid in CAD and dissection

TRIMETHAPHAN
Ganglionic blocker
Titrated with patient sitting (its activity depends on this)-has been largely replaced
In aortic dissection
Liberates histamine
Ileus, urinary retention and respiratory arrest

DIURETICS
as adjuncts

PHENTOLAMINE
If HTN due to pheochromocytoma
HTN due to tyramine ingestion by a patient on MAO inhibitors

CLONIDINE
Over several hrs
Sedation and rebound hypertension is seen

CAPTOPRIL
In 15-30 mins
Response variable

NIFEDIPINE
Rapid reduction
Unpredictable
Hypotension, reflex tachycardia
Not advised without beta blocker
May cause stroke and mi

ASYMPTOMATIC HTN
no proven benefit of rapid reduction
cerebral or MI can be induced by aggressive anti HTN therapy
goal is to reduce BP to 160/110 mmHg with oral therapy over several hrs
loop diuretics if not volume depleted
short acting CCB (esradipine or felodipine) or captopril

ISCHEMIC STROKE
Benefit to be weighed against possible worsening of ischemia

ACUTE PULMONARY EDEMA
Nitroprusside or NTG with loop diuretics
Avoid hydralazine, labetalol or other beta blockers

ANGINA AND ACUTE MI
Nitroprusside or NTG
Labetalol also effective
Hydralazine contraindicated

DISSECTING AORTIC ANEURYSM
Depends upon mean pressure, width of pulse pressure and rate of change of pressure
Aim is to decrease sbd to 100 to 120 mmhg and decrease cardiac contractility
Nitroprusside plus iv beta blocker

WITHDRAWL OF ANTI HTN MEDICATION
Due to clonidine and propranolol
Up regulation of receptors
Readminster discontinued drug
Phentolamine, labetalol or nitroprusside if necessary

INCREASE IN SYMPATHETIC ACTIVITY
Pheochoromocytoma, GBS, Post Spinal Cord Injury, Sympathetomimetic drugs (phenylpropanoamine, cocaine, amphetamines and phencyclidine) Combination of MAO with Tyramine containing foods
Beta blocker alone contraindicated
Use of Phentolamine, Labetalol or Nitroprusside.

PREGNANCY
IV Hydralazine is DOC
Alternatives are Nicardipine or Labetalol.

DIABETIC EMERGENCIES
Larisa Gamerman, MD

DIABETIC KETOACIDOSIS (DKA)

Diagnostic criteria	Cause (most common)
• Blood glucose > 250 • PH <7.30 • HCO3 <= 18 • Anion gap >12 • + urine/serum ketones	• Noncompliance • Infection • Pancreatitis • MI, CVA • Substance abuse • Pregnancy

FIRST 12-24 HRS

Insulin (regular)	. IV bolus (not a must) 15U – only if no hypoKalemia Contin. drip 0.1 U/kg/hr to decrease glucose 75-100 mg/dl/hr. Can double the dose if no response in 2-3 hrs.
Fluids (monitor and replace urine output)	Deficit 3-6 L. (except for ESRD anuric pts.) IV NS 1-2 L over first 1-2 hrs., then 1L/hr x 1hr., then 200-300 cc/hr. till deficit is corrected.(watch for CHF) Change to D5% NS when glucose <250mg/dl Continue dextrose till IV insulin stopped, anion gap <=12, and Pt. is eating.
K replacement	start replace when K< 5.5- if + urine output. Give 20 mEq/hr.
Phosphate replacement	Not routinely necessary. Can start when Phos. <0.35 mmol/L

38

	Give neutral-phos or K- phos 0.08- 0.16 mmol/kg IV over 6 hrs.
Misc	can give IV bicarbonate if PH < 6.9 & HCO3 <5
Labs	accucheck q 1 hr. BMP on admission then in 4 hrs, then PRN.
Look for cause other than noncompliance	See above

AFTER 12-24 HRS.

Insulin	Change to SQ regular insulin if anion gap <=12 or HCO3>16 but continue IV x 60 min after first SQ injection. If Pt. is still on NPO-regular insulin - ISS q4 hrs. If Pt. is eating give home dose of NPH + ISS qAC & HS, adjust NPH to blood glucose level and regular insulin required.

HYPERGLYCEMIC HYPEROSMOLAR STATE

Diagnostic criteria	Cause (most common)
• Serum osmolality > 310 mosm/kg • Blood glucose > 600 • PH > 7.30 • HCO3 > 15 • Anion gap < 14 • Urine/serum ketones (-) or small	• Noncompliance • Infection • Pancreatitis • MI, CVA • TPN/ Parenteral glucose • Trauma

Insulin (regular)	start 1hr after IV fluids 10 U IV BOLUS (IF NO HypoKalemia) then 0.1 U/kg/hr IV or 10-20 U SQ q 4 hrs-to decrease glucose by 75-100 mg/dl/hr D/C IV insulin when glucose 250-300 mg/dL Start ISS q 4-6 hrs if Pt. on NPO Start NPH + ISS q 4-6 hrs if Pt eating Some Pts. May not require insulin Tx once recovered
Fluids (monitor and replace urine output)	Deficit 8-10 L (except for ESRD anuric pts.) IV NS if pt hypotensive & oliguric, otherwise ½ NS- 4-6L over first 8-10 hrs. Start 1-2 L over 1-2 hrs, then 1 L/hr x 1 hr, then 500cc/hr x 1-2 hrs then 200-300cc/hr till deficit is corrected (Beware of CHF).
K replacement	start when K<5.5 but less aggressive than in DKA
Phosphate replacement	Can start when Phos. <0.35 mmol/L Give neutral-phos or K- phos 0.08- 0.16 mmol/kg IV over 6 hrs.
Labs	accucheck q 1 hr BMP on admission then in 4 hrs, then PRN
Miscallaneuos	DVT prophylaxis

DIALYSIS MODALITIES
Priyanka Sharma

MODALITIES AVAILABLE
Hemodialysis

Hemofiltration
Peritoneal dialysis

ACCESS
Arterio venous
Venovenous

HEMODIALYSIS
Transport process by whish a solvent passively diffuses down its concentration gradient from one fluid compartment to the other.

HEMOFILTRATION
Uses hydrostatic pressure gradient to induce the filtration or convectiion of plasma water.
Middle and small molecular wieght molecules are removed by "solvent drag".

HEMODIAFILTRATION
Combination of hemodialysis and hemofiltration.
Solute loss primarily by hemodialysis.
25% or more by hemofiltration.

DIALYSIS TECHNIQUES
CRRT
Home dialysis
In- center dialysis

CRRT
Continuous hemofiltration
Slow continuous ultrafiltration
Continuous hemodialysis
Continuous hemodiafiltration
Continuous equilibrium peritoneal dialysis

CAPD
No significant difference in survival as compared to in-center dialysis in non diabetics.
Higher survival for young diabetics
Lower survival for elderly diabetics
In patients with severe systolic dysfunction
Pretransplantation dialysis

HIGH FLUX DIALYSIS
Decreased morbidity
More long term benefits
High blood flow rates required
Requires stable cardiovascular status

PREFERENCES
Home dialysis for young, healthy, independent patients .
CAPD for independent diabetics who have sufficient manual dexterity.
CAPD or CCPD for elderly patients with unstable hemodynamics.

INDICATIONS FOR DIALYSIS
Refractory fluid overload
Hyperkalemia
Patients who require intensive nutritional support
Signs of uremia - pericarditis, neuropathy or unexplained decline in mental status
Bun exceeds 140- 150 mg/dl

COMPLICATIONS NOTED DURING HD
Hypotension
Hypertension
Cardiac arrythmias
Bio incompatibility reactions - type a or type b

GI BLEED
Lokanathan Anand, MD

UPPER GI BLEED CAUSES
Peptic ulcer disease
    1.H. Pylori
    2.NSAIDs
    3.stress
    4.increased HCl
Esophagogastric varices
Mallory-weiss tear

LOWER GI BLEED CAUSES
Diverticulosis
Angiodysplasia
Colitis
    1.Infectious colitis
    2.Ischemic colitis
    3.Inflammatory bowel disease
Neoplasm
Hemorrhoids
Radiation telangiectasia
Following biopsy or polypectomy

APPROACH TO UPPER GI BLEED
Resuscitation
Diagnostic studies
Erythromycin
Risk stratification
Acid suppression

APPROACH TO LOWER GI BLEED
Resuscitation
Diagnostic studies
1.Coloscopy
2.Radionuclide imagining
3.Angiograpy
4.Small bowel study

GENERAL PRINCIPLES OF UPPER GI BLEED
Bleeding proximal to lig of trietz
Ng lavage yields blood or coffee-ground confirms clinical diagnosis
Assess hemodynamic stability(shock, orthostatic hypertension, decreased hematocrit 6 percent or transfusion over 2 units of packed red blood cells or active bleeding
Resuscitaion

UPPER GI BLEED
pan-endoscopy is the diagnostic modality- diagnostic and therapeutic

41

erythromycin single dose given 20-120 minutes improves visibility, shorten endoscopy time, second look endoscopy
red blood cell scan
UGI barium studies CI in active setting

UPPER GI BLEED RISK STRATIFICATION
Absence of
- debilitation
- orthostatic hypertension
- sever liver disease
- severe concomitant disease
- anticoagulation therapy or coagulopathy
- voluminous hematemesis or severe melena
- severe anemia HB less than 8g/dl

UPPER GI BLEED ACID SUPPRESSION
PPI has significant reduction in rate of rebleed, hospital system need for bld transfusion in high--risk ulcer bleeder
treated with endoscopic therapy
H2 blocker have not shown any significant reduction to lower rebleed

UPPER GI BLEED TREATMENT
- Somatostatin has more effective than vasopressin-few side effects
- endoscopic therapy is treatment of choice for active variceal hemorrhage
  - banding
- 2.sclerotherapy
- Balloon tamponade -short term
- surgery - TIPS Rec if recurs within 48 hours
- Intravariceal injection of thrombin
- assess the risk of the patient

LOW RISK
Young
Maintain hematocrit above 20 percent

HIGH RISK
elderly
severe comorbidity such as CAD, cirrhosis
maintain hematocrit above 30 percent
coagulopathy-INR more than1.5 and platelet less than 50

NUTRITIONAL SUPPORT OF THE STRESSED ICU PATIENT
Hina Azmat, M.D

INJURY STRESS RESPONSE AND STARVATION
- Injury stress response: CNS mediated endocrine response with increased levels of catecholamines, steroids and glucagon, also includes SIRS with its mediators (TNF-alpha, IL-1, IL-2, IL-6), it is not clearly understood.
- ISR: Increases REE(resting energy expenditure): glucose stores followed by gluconeogenesis, then lipolysis, then protein catabolism.
- Starvation:in 72 hours,proteins r primary energy source, then fat is mobilized, if starvation continues, energy requirements decrease and protein is protected.
- Stressed ICU patient needs more non-protein calories(25kcal/kg/day) and more protein(1.3g/kg/day), may even need upto2g/kg/day
- Persistent hypercatabolism_dec muscle mass-dec visceral protein-dec organ function-dec immune response-infections-multiple organ failure
- Studies on burn and trauma patients: early nutrition preferably by enteral route improves outcome.

NOSOCOMIAL INFECTIONS
Severe SIRS – early MOF– Compensatory anti-inflammatory response syndrome (CARS)- delayed immunosuppression-secondary infection-late MOF
Immune-enhancing formula eg. Glutamine stimulates lymphocyte and monocyte functions
Dysfunctional gut: reservoir for pathogens that cause late MOF associated infections
Prospective RCT's –selective gut decontamination, early enteral nutrition,and immune-enhancing enteral formulas reduce nosocomial infections esp. pneumonia
Nutritional Assessment
History: anorexia, vomiting, diarrhea, weight loss
P. E. : muscle wasting, loss of SC fat, dermatitis, glossitis, poor wound healing.
Lab Data: Selected hepatically synthesized transport proteins like albumin, transferrin, pre-albumin, and retinol-binding protein
Anthropometric measurements: Height, weight and limb circumference (take into account edema) most useful in monitoring patients on home TPN

NUTRITION REQUIREMENTS
Harris-Benedict equation: energy requirements in fasted, resting, non-stressed state with stress multiplication factors of 1.2 to 1.6
COPD patients: diet high in glucose will produce more CO_2 and high minute ventilation and difficulty to wean, better to give more non-protein calories as fat and do not overfeed
If over- nutrition is considered the reason for difficulty to wean, cut nutrition by half day before weaning trial, if still cannot wean consider other cause like inadequate ventilatory endurance and unrecognized hypermetabolism

TPN INDICATIONS:
Massive bowel resection
High output fistula refractory to elemental diet
Unable to meet >60% of nutritional needs by ICU day 8
Malabsorption
Persistent ileus or bowel obstruction
Persistent risk for bowel necrosis

TPN
Pre-operative TPN: not good : more post-op septic complications: increased tumour burden in cancer patients
Stress-formula TPN: more AA's to prevent auto-cannibalism of proteins: specialty formulas with renal and hepatic adjusted AA's : no improvement in morbidity or mortality
Lipids-taken up by RES-inc. sepsis because of immunosuppression

COMPLICATIONS OF TPN
Overfeeding, underfeeding, specific nutrient deficiencies or toxicities
Metabolic (hyperglycemia, electrolyte, fluid, acid-base, and LFT's)
Infectious (catheter-related sepsis)
Mechanical (hemothorax, pneumothorax, subclavian vein thrombosis)
Re-feeding syndrome:rapid and excessive feeding of severely malnourished patients results in ion fluxes into cells with sudden drop of P, K, Ca, Mg: cardiac arrythmias, confusion, resp. failure and death

ENTERAL NUTRITION
Enteral route is preferred to the parenteral route.
Prevents G.I. mucosal atrophy, preserves normal gut flora and reduces septic morbidity by reducing bacterial translocation
Indications for early enteral nutrition (table 7 on pg:494)
Feed by postpyloric route early in the critical illness and by prepyloric route late in the illness
Immune-enhancing diets containing arginine, glutamine, 4-3 poly-unsaturated fatty acids and nucleotides have shown good outcomes in patients likely to suffer from major septic complications and MOF
Nonocclusive bowel necrosis is a complication of enteral nutrition

CONTROVERSIES

43

Recent trial showed increased mortality in critically ill patients who were given recombinant human growth hormone.
Jejunal feeding instead of TPN is associated with decreased septic complications
Obese patients should be fed as early as their non-obese counterparts to prevent harmful loss of their lean body mass
Formulas with decreased carbs and increased lipids may delay gastric emptying in diabetics.

INFECTIOUS DISEASES OF THE CNS
Vesselin Dimov, MD

Meningitis
Encephalitis
Abscess
Epidural abscess

MENINGITIS CAUSE = BAT
B acterial
A septic' viral
T B

Start ABx Tx imediately if you suspect meningitis' pneumococci/meningococci can kill the Pt while waiting for the CT head

SYMPTOMS
Classic
Fever
Stiff neck
Headache
Rash

Common
Photophobia
Nausea
Vomiting
Malaise
Lethargy

COMPLICATIONS
Cerebral edema
ICP/
Cerebral infarction
Brain abscess
Seizures (40% cases)
Subdural empyema
Venous Thrombosis

DIAGNOSIS
Brudzinski's sign
Kernig's sign
CT
Spinal tap
Blood culture

MG DX= DON'T MISS !!!:
M eningeal sx
I CP/ sx
S eptic sx= T F /

S pinal tap= LP, CSF

Meningitis is one of the big killers and it kills quickly
Delays for rounds or lab results could be fatal
Suspect meningitis nothing should delay prompt "blind" empiric Tx and Blood Cx x 2
Prepare for LP

LUMBAR PUNCTURE
Single most important diagnostic test
Mandatory, esp. if bacterial meningitis suspected
If LP contraindicated, obtain BCs (+ in 50-60%), then begin empirical Rx

TREATMENT
Microbial Therapy ~ 1st broad spectrum, then specific "shoot 1st and ask questions later"

Supportive Measures
Fluid replacement
Monitor and treat cardiovascular function and oxygenation
Monitor and treat ICP
Treat seizures

EMPIRIC ABX CHOICE
Increasing prevalence of PCN-resistant pneumococci' Cefotaxime 2gm Q 4hr IV or Ceftriaxone 2 gm Q 12 hr IV
A few pneumocci have resistance to 3rd gen. cephalosporins' add Vancomycine until sensitivities are available

BRAIN ABSCESS
Empiric Therapy
Ceftriaxone / Cefotaxime
Metronidazole
Vancomycin
Surgery' early aspiration recommended

VIRAL MENINGITIS
Self-limiting disease which tends to be nonfatal (<1% mortality rate)
Caused by enteroviruses (40%), the mumps virus (15%) . . . unknown in 30% of all cases
Symptoms are the same as bacterial meningitis

TYPES OF INFECTION
Diseases of the Brain and Meninges

Viral Meningitis
Rabies (pix)
Encephalitis
Herpes Meningoencephalitis
Polyomavirus

TREATMENT
Supportive treatment
Hospitalization
IV fluid replacement
Airway management
Respiratory support if needed
Prevention of 2o infections - Pneumonia, UTI, etc.
Good nursing care

References

Infectious Diseases of the CNS. Laurie Lower, 2001, ppt.
Adjunctive Dexamethasone Treatment in Patients with Bacterial Meningitis. David Malmud, 2001, ppt.

PNEUMONIA
Roomana Akthar, MD

SYMPTOMS:
URI, cough, sputum, wheezing, progressive dyspnea, fever, malaise, pleuritic chest pain, abdominal pain, nausea, vomiting, obtundation.

PREDISPOSING FACTORS:
CHF, COPD, smoking, sicklE cell disease, bronchiectasis, hypogammaglobulinemia, chnge in mental status, seizures, aspiration, immunocompromised.

SYSTEMIC:
Fever
Temp > 40 suggest bacterial source

CHEST AND SKIN FINDINGS:
Congestion, tachypnea, possible retraction, splinting, cough, hoarseness, stridor, wheezing, rhonchi, consolidation, dullness to percussion
Exanthem in the skin

MOST COMMOMN CAUSES:
Srep pneumoniae , legionella
H. Influenza, anaerobes
Viral agents , TB
Group a strep , Q- fever
Pseudomonas , Tularemia
S.aureus
E.coli
Klebsiella

IN SPECIAL CASES:
•COPD/ cigarette smoking
  h.influenza, klebsiella
•Diabetes
  klebsiella, e-coli, gram negatives
•Alcohol abuse
  klebsiella, anaerobes, gram negative, m.tub
•Sickle cell disease - salmonella
•IV drug abuse - staph aureus
•Cystic fibrosis - resistant pseudomonas

DIFFERENTIAL DIAGNOSIS:
CHF
Tumor
Pulmonary contusion
Pleural effusion
Pleral/ parenchymal thickening or scarring
Atelectasis

DIAGNOSTIC TOOLS:
CBC with diff (left shift indicates bacterial process)

46

O2 saturation / abg
CXR
Sputum for culture and gram stain
Blood/ urine for c&s
Thoracentesis

PORT SCORE:
Age male; no of years of age
        female; no of years of age – 10.
Nursing home resident: +10

Comorbid illness:
Neoplastic ; +30
Liver ; +20
Chf ; +10
Cva ; +10
Renal disease ; +10

Physical exam:
Change in mental status; +20
Respiratory rate > 30; +20
Sbp < 90; +20
Temp < 35 or > 40; +15

Labs
Art ph <7.35; +30
BUN >30; +20
Na <130 ; +20
Glucose > 250; +10
Hct < 30; +10
Art po2< 60 ; +10
Pleural effusion; +10

Risk:
Class points mortality site of care

Class	points	mortality	site of care
		0.1%	o/p
<70		0.6%	o/p
71- 90		2.8%	o/p briefi/p
91- 130		8.2%	in patient
> 130		29.2%	in patient

TREATMENT:
Strep pneumoniae
Pen g/ v, amoxicillin, macrolides, cephalosporin, doxycycline, fluroquinolone, vanco
H.infuenza
    cefotaxime / ceftriaxone, cefuroxime, doxy, arithro, bactrim
Staph
    pen g/ pen v, ceph, vanco
Mycoplasma
    erythro, doxy, azithro
Legionella
     erythro with or without rifampin, bactrim, azithr0

TREATMENT:
Chlamydia
    clarithro, cipro, doxy

47

Pcp
  bactrim, pentamidine, prednisone.
Klebsiella
  3rd gen ceph + aminoglycoside
  aztreonen/ imipenem
Pseudomonas anti pseudomonal/ betalactam+aminoglycoside
Anaerobes: clinda + metronidazole + beta lactam

PREVENTION:
Pneumococcal vaccine for:
Chronic heart or lung condition
Cirrhosis
Nephrosis
DM
Immunosuppression

COMPLICATIONS:
Pleural effusion
Empyema
Lung abscess
Septicemia
Metastatic infections
Respiratory failure
Jaundice

ONCOLOGY EMERGENCIES
Nabeel Sarhill, MD

STRUCTURAL-OBSTRUCTIVE EMERGENCIES.
Superior vena cava syndrome.
Spinal cord compression.

METABOLIC EMERGENCIES.
Hypercalcemia.
Hyperuricemia.
Hypoglycemia.
Lactic acidosis.

TREATMENT-RELATED EMERGENCIES.
Tumor lysis syndrome

SUPERIOR VENA CAVA SYNDROME
Definition: obstruction of blood flow through SVC.
Occur as manifestation of either primary or metastatic tumor, or as thrombosis due to central line.
SVCS can lead to life-threatening cerebral edema or laryngeal edema

PATHOLOGIC DIAGNOSIS OF SVCS

Histolology	Percent
Lung cancer	65
Lymphoma	8
Other Malignacies	10

Nonneoplastic	12
Undiagnosed	5

SYMPTOMS AND SIGNS OF SVCS

Symptoms	Percent
Dyspnea	63
Facial swelling	50
Cough	24
Signs	
Venous distension of neck	66
Venous distension of chest	54
Facial edema	46

DIAGNOSTIC PROCEDURES OF SVCS
Clinically.
Sputum cytology thoracocentesis.
Chest X-ray.
Chest CT.
MRI, no advantages over chest CT.

Invasive procedures.
Bronchoscope.
Percutaneous needle biopsy.
Mediastinoscope.
Thoracotomy.

TREATMENT OF SVCS
Goals
Relieve symptoms.
Cure the primary malignant process

Emergent R/T before tissue prove when respiratory compromise or CNS symptoms
Consider the histology diagnosis and stage.
Bed rest, elevate head, O_2 use.
Steroids can be used but seldom helpful (IV dexamethasone 10mg q6h for 2 days, followed 4mg oral q6h).
NSCLC: R/T or combine chemotherapy.
SCLC: chemotherapy or combine R/T.
NHL: chemotherapy remain standard.
Catheter-induced: anticoagulants and removal of catheter.
Intraluminal stenting

SPINAL CORD COMPRESSION
Hematogenous spread.
Usually in the vertebral body.

Compression of cord microvasculature by bone or tumors.
Circulatory disturbance.
Secondary change (cord edema, ischemia, or infarction).
Neurologic signs.

CLINICAL PRESENTATION OF CORD COMPRESSION(II)
Local pain(90%),constant, dull, aching, and progressive.
Weakness(80%), neurologic signs.

DIAGNOSTIC EVALUATION
Clinical signs and symptoms.
Plain radiograph detected 80% of cases.
MRI

CT
Evaluating vertebral stability and bone destruction.
Before surgical management.

TREATMENT OF SPINAL CORD COMPRESSION
Initial treatment: steroid plus radiation. And consulted neurosurgery, neurology.

Indication of surgical intervention:
Unknown diagnosis.
Spinal instability.
Failure of radiation therapy

Chemotherapy: chemosensitive tumor.

Steroid
IV dexamethasone 10mg q6h for 2 days, followed 4mg oral q6h.
Improve peaked at day 2 and diminished by day 4 and tapered every 4 days.

HYPERCALCEMIA
Correct serum calcium =measured calcium +0.8(4.0-measured albumin).

Hypercalcemia,
mild≤ 12.0mg/d.
modaret12-13.5mg/d.
severe ›13.5 mg/d.

DISEASE ASSOCIATED WITH HYPERCALCEMIA
Cancer.
Endocrine disease.
Infectious disease.
Renal insufficiency.
Drug related.
Granulomatous disease.

PATHOGENESIS
Direct bone destruction: osteolytic.

Humorally mediated.
PTH, PTH-RP.
Vit D3.
Prostaglandins.
Cytokines.

CLINICAL MANIFESTATIONS OF HYPERCALCEMIA

Category	Manifestation

General	Dehydration, weigh loss, anorexia.
Neuromuscular	Fatigue, lethargy, weakness, confusion, psychosis, seizure, coma.
GI	Nausea, vomiting, constipation.
GU	Polyuria, renal failure.
Cardiac	Bradycardia, PR, QT, wide T wave,

TREATMENT OF CANCER-RELATED HYPERCALCEMIA
General measures.
Best treatment for underlying cancer.
Increase urinary excretion.
Decrease bone resorption, inhibit osteoclast.
Encourage ambulation

Hydration and Diuretics.
IVF, NS 500cc/hr for 3-5hr
after good hydration, Furosemide 10-40 mg IV q6hr

Calcitonin.
Rapid onset (2 to 4) hrs, peak at 48 hrs, then diminish.
4 IU/Kg IV BID for 2 days.

Corticosteroids
indication
malignancy
Granulomatous diseases
vit D intoxication
hydrocortisone 200-300mg IV/day

Plicamycine
Rapid onset (12hr) hrs, with duration 3-7days
25mcg/kgin 250cc of NS infusion in 1hr
risk of hepatic and renal toxicity, bleeding and thrombocytopenia.

Bisphosphonates.
Pamidronate 60-90mg IVF 3 hrs.
Zometa 4 mg IV in 15 min can be repeated weekly

Gallium nitrate (not the radioisotope)
100-200 mg/m2/day over 24hr for up to 5 days in rehydrated nonoliguric (urine output 1500-2000 ml/day)
indication
bisphosphonates resistant

TUMOR LYSIS SYNDROME
Rapid release of intracellular contents.
Large tumor burden and exquisite chemosensitive tumor.

Hyperkalemia   →Lethal arrhythmia.

Hyperuricemia   →ARF.
Hyperphosphatemia   →ARF.
Hypocalcemia   →Cramps, tetany.

TREATMENT OF TUMOR LYSIS SYNDROME
Recognition and prevention.
Hydration 24 hrs before starting C/T.
Allopurinol, 300 mg qd.
Sodium bicarbonate, keep urine pH>7.0.
Monitor serum eletrolytes.
Consider early initiation of renal dialysis.

LEUKOSTASIS
Cellular hyperviscosity.
More common in AML than ALL
Symptoms and signs: dyspnea, hypoxia; headache, stupor, coma, and can progress to CNS hemorrhage and death.
Suspect in patients with these symptoms and blast > 50000/uL.

TREATMENT
Hydration 250-500 cc/hr for few hours.
Hydroxyurea 20-30mg/kg/dayin 2 doses.
Leukapheresis and antileukemic therapy ASAP.
whole brain XRT therapy if CNS symptoms significant
Avoid transfusion of PRBC.

PERIOPERATIVE MANAGEMENT ISSUES
Vesselin Dimov, MD

Pain
Delirium
Ischemia

PAIN
Do not forget how painful pain is.
A global approach to pain management — the WHO ladder

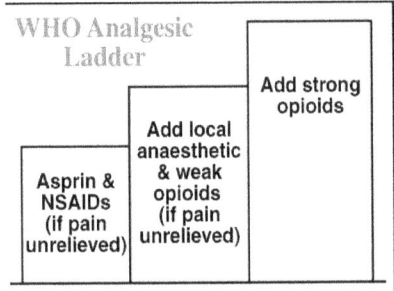

Pre-emptive analgesia in the control of pain
Pre-emptive analgesia (anticipatory pain control) is defined as "the administration of analgesic agents prior to an injury in order to prevent the development of central nervous system hyper-excitability or sensitization".

HOW DO YOU ASSESS INTERVENTIONS?
Clinical observation

Face — comfort/discomfort
Mute/withdrawn
Posture/movement
Feeding
Sleeping
Interaction with environment

DELIRIUM

DSM-IV Criteria for Delirium
Disturbance of consciousness with reduced ability to focus, sustain or shift attention
A change in cognition or development of a perceptual change not accounted for by pre-existing, established or developing dementia
The disturbance fluctuates over a short period of time and tends to fluctuate during the course of the day
Evidence in history, examination or investigation of an organic cause
(Diagnostic and Statistical Manual of Mental Disorders, 4th ed Text Revision (DSM-IV-TR). American Psychiatric Association 2000)

SPECTRUM OF PSYCHOMOTOR ACTIVITY
Hypoactive delirium (lethargy, excess somnolence, sluggish)
Hyperactive delirium (agitated, hallucinating, inappropriateness)
Mixed - combination of both

DELIRIUM: PROGNOSIS
Patients need to be followed for the development of dementia.
Following recovery, annual incidence of dementia 20%

DELIRIUM CAUSES= *MAD HIVES:*
M etabolic→ lf, cri
A lcohol withdrawal
D rug o-d
H ypoxia→ copd
I nfection
V ascular→ cva, ami
E pilepsy
S ubdural ich

MEDICATIONS ASSOCIATED WITH DELIRIUM
Any drug can potentially cause confusion.
Take a careful history of any new drug started or any old drug stopped recently.

DIFFERENTIAL DIAGNOSIS OF DELIRIUM
Communication Problem
Mood disorder (depression and severe anxiety)
Psychosis
CVA
Postictal
Dementia

DISTINGUISH DEMENTIA AND DELIRIUM
Relatively abrupt decline in cognition, function and behaviour
Change in level of consciousness
Presence of hallucinations
Presence of potential causal agent(s)

How well do we detect Delirium?

Only 30-50% have symptoms/signs documented by MD's
RN's document 60-90%

Confusion Assessment Method
Acute Change in mental status
AND
Inattention/fluctuation
PLUS
Disorganized thinking
OR
Altered level of consciousness

Sensitivity 94 - 100%
Specificity 90 - 95%
Ann Intern Med 1990; 113:941
Arch Intern Med. 1995; 155:301

DELIRIUM COGNITIVE EVALUATION
MMSE:
Inaccurate tool to diagnose delirium as the patient:
fluctuates
has poor attention/concentration

APPROACH TO DELIRIUM
Teat all precipitating causes including pain!
Optimise physiological status (hydration, nutrition etc)
Stabilise environment and re-orientate
Encourage familiar faces for reassurance e.g. family members
Avoid restraints

TREATING DELIRIUM
1. Use a single medication rather than two to decrease the potential for side effects/drug interactions.
2. Start with a low dose
3. Try to stop the medication as soon as possible, focusing on correcting the underlying cause for the delirium.
5. Non-Pharmacological Interventions.

Haldol
Try to only use for **severe** agitation
Can use used im/iv
Start with 0.5 - 1 mg initial dose, gradually titrating to a maximum of 4 mg/day
Avoid in individuals with parkinson's disease

ISCHEMIA
PERIOPERATIVE STROKES
1-6%→ cardiothoracic surgery

RISK FACTORS:
Prior CVAs
CHF
Carotid bruits
COPD
Atrial Tachyarrhythmias

SUSPECT CVA IF:
Sudden change in MS
Delay in awaking from anesthesia

Focal deficits
Urgent evaluation → CT head w/o contrast

PERIOPERATIVE AMI RISK FACTORS:
Prior CAD
CHF
Valvular disease
DM
Arrhythmias
Advanced age
Prior CVA
HTN

Perioperative meds shown to decrease AMI risk
Atenolol
Clonidine

Beta blockers contraindicated in moderate/severe asthma
NOT in COPD

LAB WORK
Cardiac surgery and other surgeries-> release CK

Troponin levels are routinely elevated after cardiac surgery to < 3 ng/mL

AMI if troponin > 10 ng/mL

References
Delirium in the Elderly. Melissa M. Stiles, 2002, ppt.
Diagnosis and management of Delirium. Shah Yogesh, 2001, ppt.

SEIZURE DISORDER
Vesselin Dimov, MD

Seizures = fire in the attic
International Classification of Epileptic Seizures
Simpleton's Seizure Classification

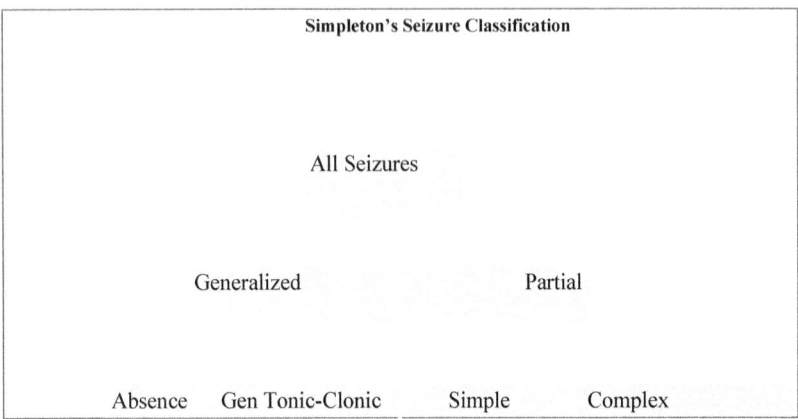

Simpleton's Seizure Classification

All Seizures

Generalized   Partial

Absence   Gen Tonic-Clonic   Simple   Complex

SEIZURES
2% of population
3% of ICU admissions

Treatment
1912→ Barbiturates
1937→ Phenytoin
1960→ BDZ

SEIZURE CAUSES
Drug withdrawal→ EtOH, any hypnosedative agent
Illicit drugs esp. cocaine
CT head→ CVA, CNS infection, TU→ 62% of ICU patients with seizures
Hypoglycemia
Rarely hypocalcemia, hypomagnesemia

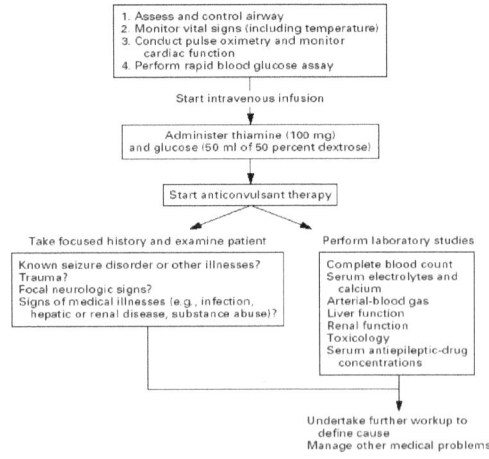

1. Assess and control airway
2. Monitor vital signs (including temperature)
3. Conduct pulse oximetry and monitor cardiac function
4. Perform rapid blood glucose assay

Start intravenous infusion

Administer thiamine (100 mg) and glucose (50 ml of 50 percent dextrose)

Start anticonvulsant therapy

Take focused history and examine patient

Known seizure disorder or other illnesses?
Trauma?
Focal neurologic signs?
Signs of medical illnesses (e.g., infection, hepatic or renal disease, substance abuse)?

Perform laboratory studies

Complete blood count
Serum electrolytes and calcium
Arterial-blood gas
Liver function
Renal function
Toxicology
Serum antiepileptic-drug concentrations

Undertake further workup to define cause
Manage other medical problems

SEIZURE WORKUP
CT head
EEG
If CNS infection suspected: CT head→ LP→ CSF→ ABx

STATUS EPILEPTICUS
Seizure activity > 20 min→ do not wait for this period to start Tx
Most seizures stop within 2-3 min→
Treat after 5 min of seizure activity or after the 2nd seizure occuring w/o recovery
Do not delay Tx to obtain EEG

STATUS EPILEPTICUS TX
Seizures due to EtOH withdrawal do not need chronic Tx and Phenytoin is not prophylactic
Start with Lorazepam 0.1 mg/kg IV x 1

Phenytoin is the 2nd choice if no response b/o ease of administration and lack of sedation→ DDx. BDZ
    20 mg/kg IV
AE: hypotension, arrhythmias→ 3 AVB

Fosphenytoin
Same drug maker
Safer→ no extravasation risk → DDx.Phenytoin
Drawback: much greater cost > Phenytoin

If no effect→ Phenobarbital
No CBZ b/o it is insoluble→ no IV/IM form
Resistant to Tx Status
Midazolam infusion→ load 0.2 mg/kg→ 0.1-2 mg/kg drip until seizure are controlled
Alternative infusion→ Propofol

References
Seizures and Epilepsy. F. Filloux, September 2002, ppt.
AEDs Available for Use in the Elderly. Leppik, 1998, ppt.
Status epilepticus. Paulo R M de Bittencourt, ppt.

SEIZURES, STROKE AND OTHER NEUROLOGICAL EMERGENCIES
Lubna Salman, MD

SEIZURE ETIOLOGY.
Anoxia.
Stroke.
Withdrawal from antiepileptic drugs.
Cryptogenic.
Related to alcohol withdrawal.
Metabolic disorders. Hypoosmolar and nonketotichyperglycemia.
CNS infection.
Trauma.
Increase risk in pt.with renal failure or altered blood-brain barrier while on imipenem-cilastatin.
Pt. receiving penicillin (GABA antagonist) are also at risk.
Transplant pt. receiving cyclosporin.

CLINICAL MANIFESTATION
Three problems occur in seizure recognition.
•Complex partial seizure in the setting of impaired awareness.

•Seizure in pt. receiving pharmacologic paralysis.
•Misinterpretation of other abnormal movements as seizures.
ICU pts. often have depressed consciousness in the absence of seizures.. A further decline in alertness may reflect seizure: an EEG is required.
Pt. receiving NMJ blockers do not menifest the usual sign of seizures.
Autonomic signs of seizure, HTN, Tachy and pupillary dilatation may also be the effects of pain or response to inadequate sedation.
So.. Pt. with these findings who have a potential for seizure should have an EEG.

DIAGNOSTIC APPROACH
HISTORY.
Observation… the most imp. Activity during a single seizure.
Drugs.. Esp.in settings of renal and hepatic insuficiency.
Alcohol, narcotic or hypnosedative… withdrawal.

PE
Evidence of cardiovascular disease or systemic infection should be sought.
Skin and fundi should be examined.
LABS
Illicit drug screening.
Electrolytes and serum osmolality.
CT OR MRI should be performed with new seizure.
CSF.
EEG.

MANAGEMENT.
Establish an airway.
Determine the BP.
    Hypo.. Fluid replacement and/vasoactive agents.
    Hyper.. no. treatment until seizure is controlled.
Rapidly determine the blood glucose…unless pt. is known norme- or hyper, give dw(1mg/   kg) and B1.
Terminate seizure.
    Lorezepam 0.1 mg/kg at 0.04mg/min. if persist,
    Phenytoin 20mg/kg at 0.3mg/kg/min. If persist
    Midazolam 0.2mg/kg ..at 0.1-2.0mg/hr. Or
    Propofol 1-3mg/k at 1-15mg/kg/hr "AT THIS STAGE PT.SHOULD BE INTUBATED. If not controlled
    Phenobarbital 12mg/kg at 0.2-0.4mg/kg/min.with EEG monitor with a goal of seizure supp."MOST PT.
    Ketamine 1mg/kg is a potent anti NMDA.(useful in refractory to GABA agonist.
Prevent recurrence.

TREAT COMPLICATIONS.
Rhabdomyolysis
Hyperthermia.
Cerebral odema.

NEUROLOGICAL EMERGENCIES

NEUROLEPTICMALIGNANT SYN
It occur in less then 1% of pt. exposed to high potency anti psychotics, but may be more frequent in pt. requiring higher than normal dose or multiple agents.

MAJOR DX FEATURES,
Fever.
Severe rigidity.
Tremor.
Optundation .

Autonomic dysfunction.

Complication:Leokocytosis, rhabdomyolysis….renal failure. DIC, pulmonary embolism, thrombocytopenia.

Managemants: DC drug, hydration, dopa agonist, dantrolene, ECT.

2.MALIGNANT HYPERTHERMIA
It is an anesthetic complication.

AD.

Abnormally high Ca release from sarcoplasmic Ca channel…lowers the threshold for sustained m's contraction.

In a typical case,

A rise in end-tidal CO2…signify MH onset.

Rapid rise in temp.

Mtabolic acidosis.

Hypoxemia.

Cardiac arrythmias

Major management issue is termination of drug and dantrolene.

SEROTININ SYNDROME.
Most pt.with SS are receiving more than 1 serotenergic agent or a MAOI, raising extracellular serotanin conc.

Although overdose of single agent may trigger the synd.

SS resemble NMS but is frequently associated with myoclonus and less with m's rigidity.

Autonomis instability is common in both .

A case of SS also involving stroke in a young pt. suggests   that the spectrum of this disorder may involve ppt.of the cmplicated migrain.

Treatment is supportive.

LETHAL CATATONIA
Often began with extreme psychotic excitation,leads to fever ,exhaustion and death.

Essentially indistinguishable from NMS, which which begans with sev. m's rigidity.

LC required neuroleptic treatment although ECT is more commonly employed.

Underlying pathophysiology remains unknown.

COMA
Raj Edula, MD

NOMENCULATURE
A state of pathological unconciousness. Pts are unaware of their environment & are unrousable.

OTHER RELATED CONDITIONS
Persistent vegetative state:

State of wake fullness without awareness

May represent a transition between   coma & recovery or coma & death.

Brain death:

Cessation of cerebral & brain stem function. ie : no respiratory drive & no central reflexes. Spinal reflexes may persist. Cardiovascular activity may persist for as long as 2 weeks

Locked in syndrome.

Conciousness is preserved. Motor output is severely restricted.

Akinetic mutism.

Medial orbitofrontal dysfunction. Awake   but complete apathy & amotivational state.

GENERAL CONSIDERATIONS
A true neurological emergency.

Result of a diverse set of medical conditions.

Simple practical approach is needed.

TWO COMPONENTS OF CONCIOUSNESS
Arousal / awakefullness
Awareness

COMPONENTS
Awakefullness:
    Ascending reticular activating system.
    Medial brain stem pathways to forebrain.
Awareness:
    Intact cerebrocortical activity. Perception & cerebral processing.

PATHOPHYSIOLOGY
Two general ways in which conciousness can be impaired.

Structural coma:
    local tissue damage. Mass lesion or compression directly damaging &impairing function of aras.
Toxic / metabolic coma
    diffuse biochemical derangement impairing function of cerebral cotex as a whole.

CAUSES
Metabolic
Drugs & toxins
Head trauma
Global ischemia
Infection
Inflammation
Hypoglycemia
DKA
Hypoxemia
Hypercapnia

Metabolic
Hyponatremia
Hypernatremia
Hypercalcemia
Liver failure
Renal failure
Thiamine deficiency
Hypertension
Seizures

Structural lesions, supra or infra tentorial.
Hemorrhage/aneurysm
Epidural / subdural hematoma
Tumor
Stroke
Venous occlusion
Abcess
Hydrocephalus

EVALUATION & MANAGEMENT
Rapid response team. Time factor.
Quick focused history.

Simultaneous intervention.

Stabilise ABC'S
Immediate routine labs
Venous access
Routine interventions, **ie**: Glucose,
thiamine, others............

HISTORY
From other individuals.
What happened? (witness)
Underlying medical problems?
Any medications used in home?
Non prescribed drug use or exposure?

EXAMINATION
Simultaneous to history.
General examination.
fever,color,bruises,odor of breath, needle tracks, signs of systemic disease.

Neurological examination.
Level of conciousness (GCS)
Evidence of impending herniation?
Brainstem function?
Any helpful focal findings?

Neurological examination
Carried out without Pt co operation.
Relies on reflex pattern and passive tone.
Level of conciousness (GCS)
Cranial nerves.
Motor tone, response &reflex pattern.
Sensory respones.

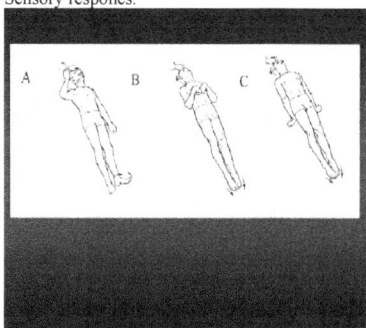

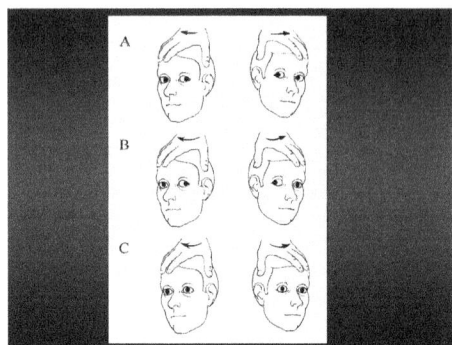

ALGORITHM TO MANAGEMENT

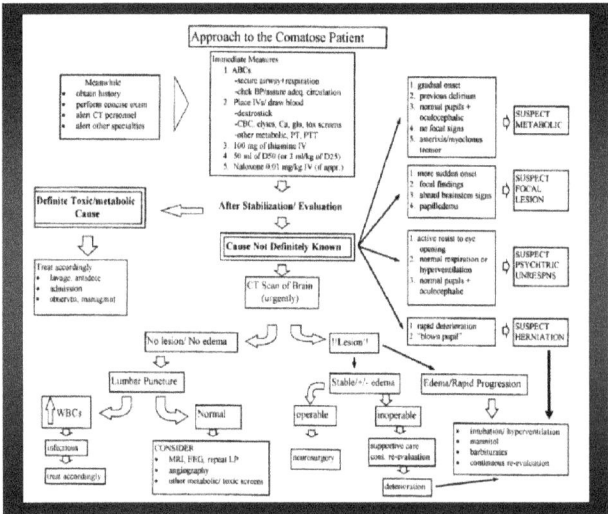

SEIZURE DISORDERS
Raj Edula, MD

DEFINITIONS

Seizure: Seizure is an event characterized by excessive or over synchronized discharges of neurons.

Epilepsy: Is a disorder characterized by recurrent seizures, not due to an immediate external cause.

Aura: Subjective disturbance of perception representing a focal electrical disturbance.

Post ictal: Period after the seizure with temporary neurological dysfunction.(Can last from few seconds to many days.)

COMMON CAUSES
Primary neurological disorders
Febrile convulsions
Idiopathic epilepsy
Trauma (head)
Stroke & vascular mal
Mass lesion
Meningitis & encephalitis
HIV encephalopathy

Systemic disorders
Hypoglycemia
Hyponatremia
Hyperosmolar states
Hypercalcemia
Uremia
Hepatic encephalopathy
Porphyria
Drug overdose
Drug withdrawl
Global cerebral ischemia
Hypertensive encephalopathy
Eclampsia
Hyperthermia

DIFFERENTIAL DIAGNOSIS
REM behaviour disorders
TIA
Transient global amnesia
Migraine
Syncope
Arrhythmias
Vertigo
Narcolepsy
Tics
Tourette syndrome

INTERNATIONAL CLASSIFICATION
Partial seizures
Simple partial seizures (conciousness not impaired)
Complex partial seizures(conciousness impaired)
Partial seizures with secondary generalization

Generalized seizures
Grand mal seizure (tonic clonic seizures)
Petit mal seizure (absence seizures)
Myoclonic seizure
Clonic seizure
Tonic seizure
Atonic seizure

Unclassified seizures
Grandmal Seizures
Classic epilepsy described since biblical times.
Begins with rigidity. (tonic phase)
Followed by repetitive clonic activity of all extremities.

63

Oral frothing, respiratory distress, cyanosis & incontinence may accompany the event.

Petit mal Seizures
Brief loss of conciousness(5-10 Seconds) without loss of postural tone.
Motor manifestations like eye blinking, head turn & automatism which is rare.
Full orientation returns promptly after seizure ends.
Usually begins before 5 years of age.
Classic EEG finding(3/S spike and wave pattern.)

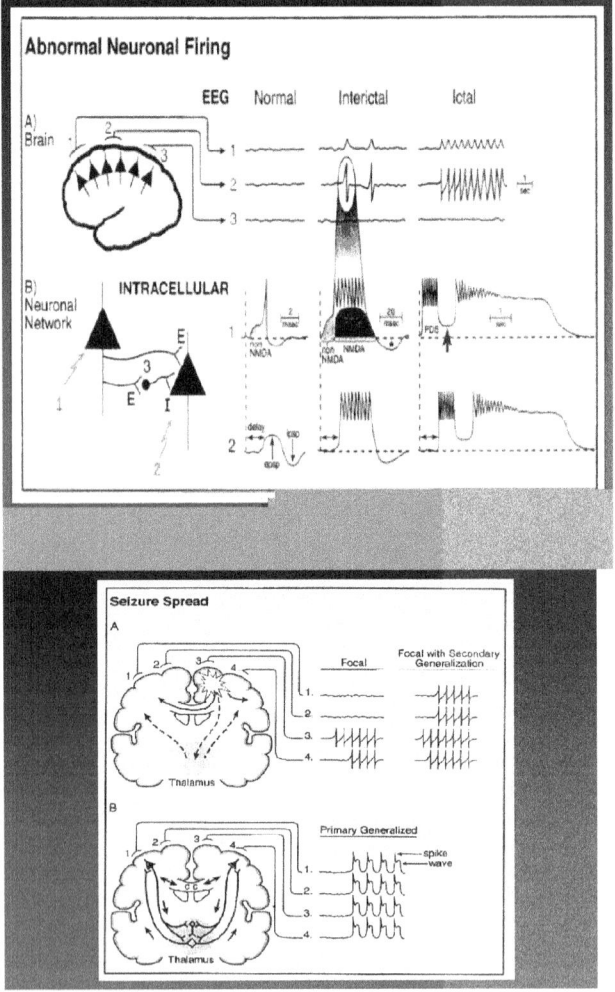

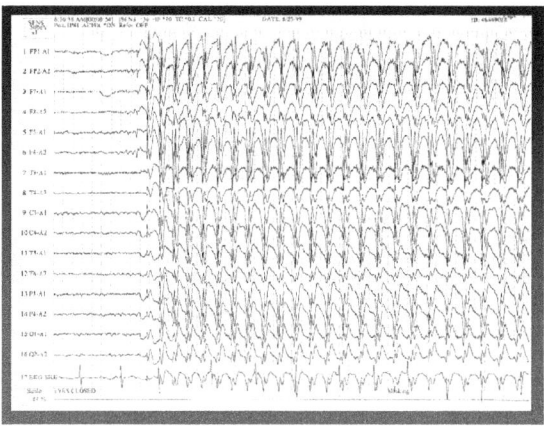

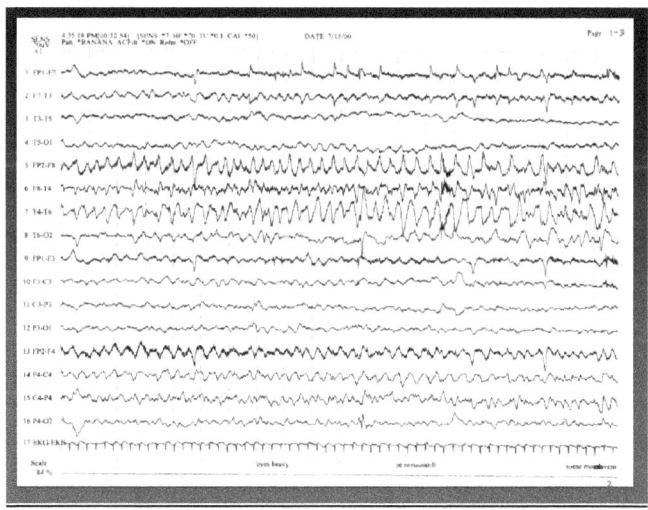

65

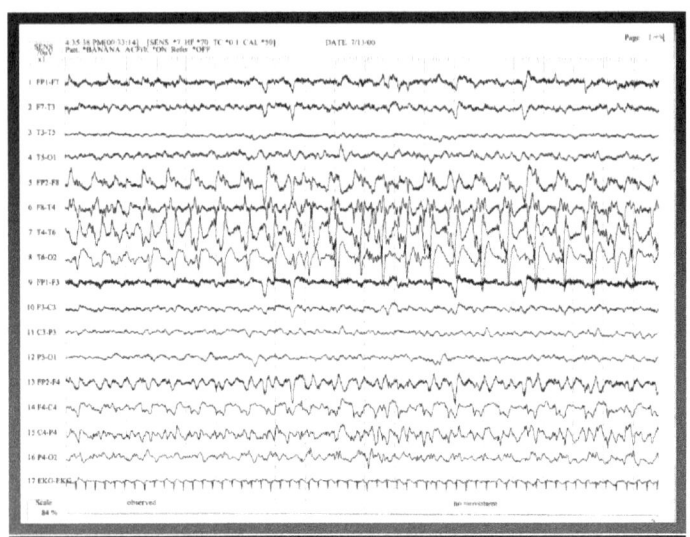

EVALUATION OF SEIZURE
History
Examination
Routine labs
Eeg
Neuro imaging
Differential diagnosis

EXAMINATION
Neurological examination is often normal.
Look for tell tale signs of seizure.
tongue laceration, lip biting, bruises, rug   *burns, babinski sign, asymmetrical motor signs.*
Cutaneous manifestations.
General examination.

NEURO IMAGING
MRI vs CT
Depends on circumstances
MRI if time permits
CT in acute setting, when LP or urgent info needed
    If blood is suspected
    Small infants

STATUS EPILEPTICUS
At least 30 minutes of continuous seizure activity, or repetitive seizure for that time, without regaining conciousness in between.
Presenting problem in 1/3 rd of pts with first onset seizure.
Beyond 60 minutes causes severe permanent brain damage or death.
Medical emergency.

MANAGEMENT OF STATUS EPILEPTICUS

66

ICU setting
Rationale: Stop the convulsion & prevent brain damage
Identify triggers
Protect patient from injury
ABC'S
IV line
Labs(CBCD, CMP, Mg, glucose, AED levels)
ABG'S
Tox screen
LP when indicated
EEG
CT

RX IN STATUS EPILEPTICUS
Lorazepam: 0.1mg/kg ,up to 4mg, may repeat q 10-15 minutes.
If continues: Phenytoin, iv, 15-20mg/kg, upto 1gm. Infuse at 3mg/kg/min. Not more than 50mg /min.
If continues: Consider intubation
Phenobarbitone
Paralytic agents

TREATMENT (WHEN TO TREAT !)
Recurrent seizures
Single seizure with high risk of recurrence.
Disease or EEG predicts recurrence.
Seizure occurs often enough or of long duration.
Seizure causes morbidity.
Interferes with function.
Creates risk.
Affects self image or well being.

DRUGS YOU MUST KNOW
Phenytoin(Dilantin)
Valproate(Depakote)
Carbamazepine(Tegretol)
Etosuximide
Phenobarbital
ACTH(Used only in infantile spasms)
Gabapentin(Neurontin)
Topiramate
Levitracetam
Lamotrigine and Vigabatrin

RX WHAT TO USE
Generalised vs Partial

Partial : Carbamazepine or Phenytoin
Valproate an option.

Generalised
Absence: Ethosuximide or Valproate
Tonic-Clonic: Valproate, Carbamazepine or
Phenytoin

DRUGS: SIMPLE RULES
Phenytoin & Carbamazepine
More or less interchangeable

Same mechanism of action.(stabilise Na channels.)
Equally effective.
Usually in partial seizures & some generalised seizures.

Valproate & Ethosuximide
Not interchangeable.
Equally effective in absence seizures.
Ethosuximide not effective for tonic-clonic seizures.

TREATMENT: GENERAL RULES
Use drug of choice.
Single agent whenever possible.
Increase dose to lowest effective dose & least amount of side effects.
Increase dose until efficacy is achieved or until unacceptable side effects occur.

PSYCHOLOGICAL CONSIDERATIONS
Newly diagnosed pts may suffer a number of losses including:
Loss of independence
Employment
insurance
Ability to drive
Self esteem
Psychological issues should be explored & appropriate referrals for help & councelling initiated.

OTHER THERAPEUTIC OPTIONS
Surgery: Resection of epileptogenic tissue.
Transcranial Magnetic Stimulation.
Complementary therapies: Herbal medicines.

WITHDRAWING AED'S
Depends on several factors.
No way to identify who will remain seizure free after withdrawl.
2 studies comparing continued Rx vs stopping.
1013 pts with epilepsy, seizure free for atleast 2 years were assigned.

Results: 78% remained seizure free continuing
Rx & 59% of those who discontinued
Rx remained seizure free.

FACTORS ASSOCIATED WITH INCREASED RISK OF RECURRENCE.
Identifiable brain disease.
Onset after age 10 to 12 years.
Poor initial response to Rx.
More than one AED at the time of withdrawl.
Specific syndromes.
Abnormal EEG's(only children)
Multiple seizure types.
Mental retardation.
Family history of epilepsy.
Abnormal neurological examination.

INFORMATION ABOUT SOME AED'S

Drugs	Frequency of dosing	Therapeutic levels (mcg)	Oral loading maintenance
Phenytoin	QD or BID	10 to 20	15 mg/kg in 3 divided doses. 5mg/kg/day maintai
Carbamazepine	BID,TID or QID	4 to 12	Start at 2-3mg/kg/d Increase every 5days Max 15-20mg/kg/day
Valproate	BID or TID	50 to 150	15mg/kg/day in 3 doses. Increase by 5 to 10mg/kg/day every week as needed
Gabapentin	TID	None	300mg 1st day, 300mg BID 2nd day 300mg TID 3rd day Max 1800mg/day

INCREASED INTRA-CRANIAL PRESSURE
Lok Anand, MD

PHYSIOLOGY
IC pressure 15 mmhg
Abnormal ICP- more than 20mmhg
Fixed internal volume –1400-1700ml.
brain parenchyma-80 percent.
CSF-10 percent.
blood-10 percent
CSF-produce by choroid plexus at rate 20ml/hr(500ml/hr). Reabsorbed via arachnoid granulation in venous system
Cerebral blood flow increase with Hypercapnia and hypoxia

Cerebral Perfusion Pressure
     CPP=MAP-ICP(50-100 mmhg)
Auto regulation-cerebral blood flow is normally maintained by cerebral vascular resistance-more than 120 mmhg
Set point for auto regulation is changed in chronic conditions-Chr. HTN
Ultimately, global or local reduction in CBF are responsible for the clinical manifestation of elevated ICP

CLINICAL MANIFESTATION
Headache-pain fibers of CN 5
Depressed global consciousness-mass effect mid brain reticular formation
Vomiting
Cushing's triad-bradycardia, res depression,HTN
Papilledema and congestion-CN 6
Focal symptoms
Kernohan'snotch phenomenon-contra lateral pupillary dilatation and ipsilateral weakness.

ICP MONITORING
Purpose is to improve the ability to maintain the adequate CPP and oxygenation.
Only way to determine CPP is to continuously monitor both ICP and BP
CPP should be kept more than 50 mmhg and ideally more than 70mmhg
Critical level is more than 110 mmhg

INDICATION FOR ICP MONITORING
•Close head trauma
•Stroke
•Intracranial hemorrhage

•Hepatic encephalopathy
•Hydrocephalus
•Subarachnoid hemorrhage
•Comatose head injury with Glasgow coma sore 3 to 8 and with abnormal cranial findings on CT scan.
•Comatose patient with normal CT scan have lower incidence of elevated ICP unless they have following features at admission
•Age more than 40
•Unilateral or bilateral motor posturing
•SBP less than 90

COMPLICATION OF ICP MONITORING
CNS infection
Intra-cranial Hemorrhage

TYPES OF ICP MONITORING
Intraventricular
Intraparenchymal
Subarachnoid
Epidural
Noninvasive and metabolic systems
Tissue resonance analysis
Transcranial doppler

MANAGEMENT OF ICP
•Resuscitation-support oxygenation, BP and end-organ perfusion

•Care should be taken to minimize further elevation of ICP during intubation through careful positioning ,appropriate choice of paralytic agents and adequate sedation-pretreatment with lidocaine

•Large shift in blood pressure should be minimized, particularly avoiding hypo tension

Emergent situation
• Life saving measures prior to detailed work-up or ICP monitoring
• In addition to standard resus
• Head elevation
• Hyperventilation to a PCO2 of 26 to 30 mmhg

TREATMENT

• ICP monitoring is associated with decreased mortality in patient with traumatic brain injury
• Goal ICP less than 20 mmhg, CPP more than 70 mmhg
• Intervention should be utilized only when ICP elevated above 20 mmhg for more than 5 to 10 minutes
• Fluid management
• Avoid all free water- D5Q,0.45 S, entral free water
• Serum osmolality should be kept more than 280 mosm/l
• Value of colloid compared to crystalloid fluid resuscitation –inconclusive
• Hyponatremia is common in elevated ICP,esp. subarachnoid hemorrhage

SEDATION
Sedation can decrease ICP by decreasing the metabolic demand, ventilator asynchrony, venous congestion and sympathetic response of HTN and tachycardia.
Propafol commonly used b/c short half life

BLOOD PRESSURE

HTN should be treated when CPP more than 120 and ICP more than 20 mmhg

POSITION
Should be positioned to maximize venous outflow from the head
Reducing excessive flexion or rotation of the neck, avoiding restrictive neck taping and minimizing stimuli that could induce Valsalva response, such as endotracheal suctioning
Head elevated 30degree above the heart to increase venous outflow.

Metabolic demand
Elevated metabolic demand in the brain increase the cerebral blood flow.

Fever-Tylenol and mechanical cooling

Seizure –Anticonvulsant should be instituted if seizures are suspected
Barbiturate sedation and hypothermia may reduce ICP-considered in refractory intracranial hypertension

Specific therapies
•Removal of mass lesion or CSF

•Osmotherapy- mannitol 20percent given as a bolus of 1gm/kg. repeat dose 0.25 to 0.5gm/kg given every 6 to 8 hours. Effects are usually present within minutes, peak at about one hour and last 4 to 24 hours. Useful parameters to monitor include serum sodium, serum osmolarity and renal function

SPECIFIC THERAPIES - CORTICOSTERIOD
Corticosteriod- not useful in management of elevated ICP from infarction, hemorrhage or head trauma.
May have a role in increased ICP caused by brain tumor and some infection

SPECIFIC THERAPIES - HYPERVENTILATION
•Hyperventilation-to lower $PaCO_2$ to 26 to 32 mmhg-rapidly decreases ICP through vasoconstriction and volume of intracranial blood. 1 mmhg change in $PaCO_2$ is associate with 3 percent change in CBF.
•Effect of hyperventilation is short-lived .
•Should not be used on chronic basis. Should be minimized in patient with traumatic brain injury or acute stroke.

SPECIFIC THERAPIES - BARBITURATES
•Barbiturates-reduces brain metabolism and cerebral blood flow.
•Continuous EEG monitoring is generally used. EEG burst suppression is an indication of maximal dosing.
•Barbiturate therapy can be complicated by hypo tension
•It requiring accurate ICP, hemodynamic, often EEG monitoring and loss of neurological examination.

SPECIFIC THERAPIES - THERAPEUTIC HYPOTHERMIA
•Therapeutic hypothermia-decreases cerebral metabolism and may reduce CBF and ICP.
•Systemic side effects-cardiac arrhythmias, severe coagulopathy
•This is limited to refractory to other therapies and clinical trial
Specific therapies - Decompressive craniectomy
•Decompressive craniectomy-improves outcome in trauma, stroke and subarachnoid hemorrhage.

Death
Jennifer Raroque, MD

OUTLINE
Historical Perspective

Review of Brain, Heart and Lung Functions
Definition of Death
Criterion of Death
Tests of Death
the Apnea Breath Test
After Diagnosing Brain Death...

CRITERIA AND TESTS OVER THE LAST FEW CENTURIES:
Unconscious
No pulse
Not breathing
With a mirror before the nose, there was no condensation formed
Pupils were fixed

Not universally accepted

HISTORICAL PERSPECTIVE
Old folks' tales
Corpses reviving during funerals
Exhumed skeletons clawed on coffin lids
Led to coffins with escape mechanisms and speaking tubes
Led to legislation requiring delay before burial

Invention of the stethoscope
It's use by a well-trained physician, together with other clinical measures laid to rest public fears of premature burial

Other inventions: EEG, EKG
More sophisticated ways of determining death

THE BRAIN
- Cerebrum- higher center; controls thought, memory, feeling, calculation, abstraction, reasoning
- Brainstem- lower center; controls spontaneous, vegetative function such as swallowing, yawning, sleep-wake cycles
- Cognition and Consciousness mediated by both

BRAIN AND LUNGS
- medulla in brainstem
- stimulate diaphragm and intercostal muscles for respiration
- adjust respiratory rate to correct levels of serum O_2 and CO_2
- destruction of these centers stops respiration > deprives heart of O_2 causing it to stop functioning

THE HEART
- Can pump blood without external control
- Brain- modulates inherent rate and force of heartbeat but are is not required for the heart to contract at a level of function that is ordinarily adequate
- If intact, even without normal brain function, will continue to beat (for 1 week in adults, 2 weeks in children) so long as:
- it receives adequate O_2
- plasma environment is within normal limits
- blood pressure is maintained

VITAL SIGNS
Reflect the interdependence of respiration, circulation and the brain
Used to diagnose death

LOSS OF VARIOUS BRAIN FUNCTIONS
4-6 minute loss of bloodflow damages the cerebral cortex
Persistent vegetative state; persistent non-cognitive state
Can have spontaneous involuntary movements- yawns, grimaces, opens eyes, breaths without respirator
10-15 minutes loss of bloodflow, the brainstem will also completely cease functioning
Continued function is possible through machines and medications

ARTIFICIAL RESPIRATOR AND OTHER LIFE SUPPORT SYSTEMS
Compensate for the inability of the thoracic muscles to fill lungs with air
Regulate rate and depth of breathing
Gas exchange continues and appropriate levels of O2 and CO2 can be maintained
Provide great benefit in avoiding irreversible harm to pt's injured heart, lung or brain
Carries a patient through period of acute need

BUT
Artificial Life Support
These new techniques have thrown a new light on the interrelationship of these organ systems
Partial brain impairment must be distinguished from complete and irreversible loss of brain function or "whole brain death"

DEFINITION OF DEATH
It's ordinary meaning should be explicit

For philosophical purposes (tests and criterion are medical)
Process rather than an event following degenerative and destructive changes in the tissues of an organism around the time of irreversible cessation or spontaneous ventilation and circulation
Necrosis of brain cells> necrosis of other vital organ cells> cooling > rigor mortis> dependent lividity> putrefaction

Stipulation of any particular point in this process as a moment of death is arbitrary
Permanent cessation of functioning of the organism as a whol- highly complex interaction of its organ systems
Permanent loss of cognition and consciousness
Therefore, persons who are in a permanent vegetative state are alive but no longer living persons and it is morally justifiable to allow them to die by discontinuing "ordinary and routine care"

CRITERION OF DEATH
Should have NO false-positives and minimal false-negatives

Criterion...
Permanent loss of cardiopulmonary function
Process of bodily disintegration follows
With artificial life support however, this criteria has become more difficult to determine

Criterion
- Total and Irreversible Loss of Whole Brain Functioning- cerebrum and brainstem
- lost consciousness, cognition
- lost respiratory drive
- lost brainstem reflexes
- lost eye movements

TESTS OF DEATH
Should never yield a false-positive result
Should produce few and relatively brief false-negatives

Tests...
1. Cessation of Heartbeat and Ventilation
        - a good and reliable test in cases not

complicated by artificial life support
- for those on life support, get lots of false negatives for 1-2 weeks
Tests...
2. Irreversible Cessation of Whole Brain Functioning
In the absence of drug intoxication, hypothermia, acute metabolic or endocrine derangement
loss of brainstem function produces loss of breathing and vasomotor control>>> apnea and hypotension

Tests
The following represent loss of whole brain function
deep coma; no motor response to painful stimuli
Absent brainstem reflexes
pupils: no light reflex, fixed dilated, anisocoria
ocular movements: (-) doll's eyes, (-) ice calorics
facial sensation and motor response- corneals, grimace
Apnea and the Apnea Breath Test

THE APNEA BREATH TEST
Jennifer Raroque, MD
Basis: PCO_2 levels of greater than 60 provides maximal stimulation for the brainstem
ABT

PRE-REQUISITES
1) core temperature greater than or equal to 36.5C
2) SBP >90mmHg
3) euvolemia
4) eucapnea (PCO_2 >/=40mmHg)
5) normoxemia (arterial PO_2 >/= 200mmHg)
6) there is a pathology to make us suspect brain death

ABT
Testing:
Disconnect the ventilator
Deliver 100% O_2 at 6LPM (hypoxia can cause arrhythmia, hypotension)
Look for respirations (thoracic excursions that produce adequate tidal volumes)
ABG after 8 minutes and reconnect the ventilator

ABT
- If during the tests, there are respiratory movements, ABT is negative (no death) and test should be repeated
- If on ABG, arterial PCO_2 is =/>60mmHg or >20 from baseline PCO_2, apnea test is positive (clinical diagnosis of brain death is made)
- ABT
- if no respiratory movements are observed, PCO_2 is < 60 and there is no cardiac arrhythmia or hypotension, repeat test disconnecting ventilator for 10 minutes

ABT
- if during testing, pt has hypotension or arrhythmia, collect ABG and then reconnect ventilator:
- if PCO_2 >/=60 or is increased 20 mmHg from baseline, ABT is positive (pt is brain dead)
- if PCO_2 </=60 or is less than 20 mmHg raised from the baseline, test is indeterminate>>> need to do confirmatory tests

CONFIRMATORY TESTS
EEG
Transcranial Doppler Ultrasonography
Angiography
Somatosensory evoked potential

AFTER DIAGNOSING BRAIN DEATH...
- family should be told in unequivocal terms that the patient died
- mechanical ventilation, fluids and BP meds are administered only to procure organs in the event that permission for this is granted
- refusal by family members to harvest organs removes the rationale for supportive therapy
- mechanical ventilation is discontinued after family has been given enough time for consideration and visitation

THROMBOCYTOSIS
Blazenka Skugor M.D.

Thrombocytosis
- Normal platelet count 150,000-450,000
- Cause:
- Extreme thrombocytosis
- Platelet count $\geq 1000,000/\mu L$
- Reactive thrombocytosis more frequent cause
- Infection, postsplenectomy or hyposplenism, malignancy, trauma, inflammation, blood loss, rebound thrombocytosis (following drug or alcohol associated thrombocytopenia)

DIFFERENTIAL DIAGNOSIS
Reactive thrombocytosis (rt)
Autonomous thrombocytosis (at)
- myeloproliferative disorders are clonal stem cell disorders that are not malignant (yet)
Polycythemia vera (PCV)
Chronic Myelogenous Leukemia (CML)
Myelofibrosis with Myeloid Metaplasia (MMM)
Essential thrombocythemia (ET)

SYMPTOMS / COMPLICATIONS
Vasomotor – headache, visual symptoms, lightheadness, atypical chest pain, acral dysesthesia,erythromelalgia (burning pain of the hands and feet with erythema)
Thrombotic complications – strokes,TIA, PE, hepatic or portal vein thrombosis, DVT etc.
Bleeding – risk increased with plt $\geq$ 1million, use of aspirin and NSAIDs

REACTIVE THROMBOCYTOSIS / CAUSES
Infection ("poor men sed rate")
Postsurgical status
Trauma
Malignancy
Postsplenectomy state
Acute blood loss or iron deficiency
Inflammation (noninfectious), RA etc.

Reactive thrombocytosis is **NOT** associated with increased bleeding, thrombosis (very rarely) or splenomegaly

DIAGNOSIS
Comprehensive history, physical exam
Labs – CBC, peripheral blood smear, serum ferritin, CRP,Howell-Jolly bodies (nuclear fragments on peripheral smear in pt with hyposplenism)

If reactive process has been ruled out, next step is to define one of myeloproliferative or myelodysplatic disorders (chronic thrombocytosis, normal iron stores, intact spleen)

WHAT NEXT?
  Bone marrow examination with reticulin staining and cytogenetic studies

CHRONIC MYELOGENEOUS LEUKEMIA (CML)
Leukocytosis
Low leukocyte alkaline phosphatase
Splenomegaly
Philadelphia chromosome(9/22 translocation) in ≥ 95%
Therapy – hydroxyurea or alpha interferon

POLYCYTHEMIA VERA
Increased RBC mass
Mild granulocytosis
Thrombocythemia
Normal oxygen saturation
Low erythropoietin levels
Older pt, pruritus after bathing, plethora of the face
Splenomegaly
Elevated leukocyte alkaline phosphastase
Complications – thrombosis, bleeding
Treatment – phlebotomy, hydroxyurea

MYELOFIBROSIS WITH MYELOID METAPLASIA
Also called agnogenic myeloid metaplasia
Splenomegaly (huge), 50% also hepatomegaly
Anemic ,poikilocytosis, megakaryocyte fragments (abnormal giant plt)
Bone marrow – increased reticulin fibers
Therapy – hydroxyurea and alkylating agents (could cause acute leukemia)

ESSENTIAL THROMBOCYTHEMIA
Platelets 600,000 to 4 million
Megakaryocytic hyperplasia on bone marrow
Diagnosis of exclusion from the other types of myeloproliferative syndrome and from reactive thrombocytosis
Chronic nonreactive thrombocythemic state
Main complications – bleeding, thrombosis
Therapy – hydroxyurea, anagrelide (Agrylin), alpha interferon

ESSENTIAL THROMBOCYTHEMIA/PROGNOSIS
Low Risk For Thrombotic Complication
  -age < 60
  -no previous history of thrombosis
  -plt < 1,500,000
  -no other risk factors
High Risk
  -age ≥ 60
  -previous history of thrombosis

MANAGEMENT OF THROMBOCYTOSIS
Bleeding – stop plt antiaggregating agent (aspirin etc.), work up for DIC and coagulation factor deficiency, endoscopic or radiologic evaluation, treatment with iron

Thrombosis – reactive thrombocytosis does not require specific treatment (very rarely cause)
  - immediate plt apheresis (>800,000)
  - plt lowering agent to keep plt <400,000

Thrombosis

- work up for additional disorder (protein C and S, antithrombin, anticardiolipin Ab, pl homocysteine, factor V and II)
- anticoagulation therapy

Vasomotor symptoms
- low dose aspirin

DIC
Priyanka Sharma, MD

CLINICAL FORMS
Acute DIC
Exposure to large amounts of tissue factor over a short period of time.
Control and compensatory mechanisms do not have enough time to recover.
Chronic DIC
Continuous or intermittent exposure to small amounts of tissue factor.
Liver and bone marrow are able to replenish the depleted coagulation proteins and platelets, respectively.

CLINICAL PRESENTATION
Acute DIC
- Bleeding (64%)
- ARF(25%): due to microthrombosis of afferent arteriole (cortical ischaemia), hypotension and/or sepsis (ATN).
- Hepatic dysfunction(19%)
- Pulmonary disease(16%): microthrombosis can worsen lung injury assoc.. with ARDS.
- CNS involvement(2%)
- Ac. promyelocytic leukemia: at time of diagnosis or at initiation of therapy. Induction of tumor cell differentiation with all-trans-retinoic acid can lead to rapid improvement.

Chronic DIC
Minor skin and mucosal bleeds
Trousseau's Syndrome
Digital ischaemia
Renal infarction
Stroke
Marantic (non bacterial thrombotic) endocarditis
Associated with solid tumors

DIAGNOSIS
Acute DIC
History of sepsis, trauma or malignancy.
Clinical presentation.
Moderate to severe thrombocytopenia (<100,000/microL).
Microangiopathic changes on peripheral blood smear.
Laboratory studies.

Chronic DIC
Platelet count moderately reduced.
Plasma fibrinogen normal or slightly elevated.
PT and PTT may be within normal limits.
Microangiopathy on peripheral smear.
Increased levels of FDPs, particularly D-dimer.

LABORATORY TESTS
FDP or D-Dimer
DIC unlikely if no evidence of accelerated fibrinolysis.

D-dimer is more specific although somewhat less sensitive than a latex agglutination test for FDPs.

Prothrombin Time
Reflects extrinsic and common pathways (Factors V, VII, X and prothrombin). These are most frequently affected.
May be normal in some patients, particularly those with abruptio placentae.

Activated PTT
Intrinsic and common pathways (Factors VIII, IX, XI, XII)

Plasma fibrinogen conc.
Low in acute decompensated DIC but may be elevated as an acute phase reactant in certain conditions (pregnancy).
Significant decrease from baseline rather than absolute value is more important.

Others
- Thrombin time- prolonged.
- Reptilase time- prolonged.
- Specific assays of Factors V, VIII and fibrinogen.
- Antithrombin (AT)- Marked reduction in levels at the onset of sepsis is an unfavorable prognostic marker.
- Protein C- reduced.
- Protein S- reduced.
- Soluble fibrin monomers- elevated in DIC and pre DIC.
High degree of sensitivity and specificity.
Specific assays are not generally available.

DIFFERENTIAL DIAGNOSIS
Severe liver disease.
Decreased synthesis of coagulation factors and inhibitors.
Thrombocytopenia due to hypersplenism.
Assoc. With chr. Or intermittent fibrinolysis,
Fibrinogenolysis and elevated levels of fdps..

Primary fibrinolysis.
Plasmin is generated in the absence of thrombosis.
Rare, but may occur with direct infusion of thrombolytic
Agents and prostate surgery.
Distinguished from DIC by absence of elevated D-dimer.

TTP-HUS
Results from primary platelet activation.
Have thrombocytopenia and microangiopathic blood
Smear.
Normal levels of coagulation components.
Little or no prolongation of pt and ptt.
Clinical setting assoc. With dic absent.
Differentiation from dic very important as it is treated
With plasma exchange which may be life saving.

TREATMENT
Correction of underlying disease.
Hemodynamic support.
Specific therapy for coagulopathy with blood component replacement therapy or heparin.
antifibrinolytic therapy, such as epsilon-aminocaproic acid (EACA) or aprotinin, is generally **contraindicated**.

SPECIFIC THERAPY
FFP- serious bleeding with/without elevated INR.

At high risk for bleeding (eg.after surgery).
Requiring invasive procedures.

Platelet Transfusion
Marked thrombocytopenia (<20,000) or moderate
Thrombocytopenia (<50,000) with serious bleeding.
1-2 units/10kg/day.
Show less than expected rise in count.

Cryoprecipitate
For fibrinogen conc. <50mg/dl.
Preferable to keep levels >100mg/dl.

Heparin
- no controlled trials indicating benefit.
- potential aggravation of bleeding.
- likely to have reduced affect due to low levels of AT.
- limited to those with chronic, compensated DIC with predominant thrombotic manifestations, those with retained dead fetus and hypofirinigenemia prior to induction of labor (septic abortion), those with excessive bleeding due to giant hemangioma and aortic aneurysm (prior to resection), and those with mismatched transfusion.
- adjunct in DIC with acute promyelocytic leukemia. However, it generally responds to all-trans retinoic acid.
- important to be sure that AT levels are 80-100% of normal.
- bolus to be avoided.
- aPTT aim of 45 seconds.
- once there is evidence of benefit, replacement therapy with FFP and cryoprecipitate is pursued.
- low molecular weight heparins also efficacious.

Protein C Concentrate
Benefit in "purpura fulminans" due to homozygous or
Acquired protein c deficiency.
Giving ffp as a source is difficult because of short half
Life in plasma.

Antithrombin
Low levels at the onset of septic shock is a sensitive
Marker for poor prognosis.
Has anticoagulant and anti-inflammatory properties.
Conflicting evidence regarding benefit.

Activated Protein C
Drotrecogin alfa (Xigris)
has both anticoagulant and anti-inflammatory properties.
directly modulates endothelial cell gene expression patterns.
greater benefit in most acutely ill patients.
evidence is conflicting regarding benefit.

BLOOD TRANSFUSIONS
Priyanka Sharma, MD

CRITERION FOR TRANSFUSIONS
- The 1988 National Institutes of Health Consensus Conference on Perioperative RBC transfusions suggested that no single criterion should be used as an indication for red cell component therapy.
- Aim is to maintain adequate "Oxygen Delivery".

- DO2=CO [(1.39*[Hb]* art oxygen saturation)
- +(PaO2 * 0.0031)]

PHYSIOLOGY OF OXYGEN UTILIZATION
- An elevated arterial lactate, oxygen extraction ratio of >0.3 and a DO2 of <10-12 ml/kg/min are each indicators of poor tissue perfusion.
- The rate of delivery of oxygen normally exceeds the consumption by a factor of 4.
- Thus, O2 delivery is adequate till Hct falls <10%, due to increased CO, right shift of O2-Hgb dissociation curve and increased O2 extraction

GUIDELINES FOR VOLUME REPLACEMENT IN ADULTS.
BASED ON LOST BLOOD VOLUME:
- >40% loss (>2000 ml) : rapid volume replacement including RBC transfusion.
- 30-40% loss (1500-2000 ml) : rapid volume replacement with crystalloids & synthetic colloids. RBC transfusion probably.
- 15-30% (800-1500 ml) : crystalloids & synthetic colloids. RBC transfusion unlikely unless co- morbidities overlap.
- <15% (<750 ml) : no need for transfusion unless co-morbidities prevail.

NEED BASED ON HEMOGLOBIN CONC.
- >10 : RBC transfusion not indicated.
- <7 : RBC transfusion indicated. If otherwise stable, give 2 units PRBCs, reassess Hgb and clinical status.
- 7-10 : correct strategy unclear.
- High risk patients (>65 yrs, CV or Resp disease) : transfused when Hgb <8.

British Committee for standards in Hematology, Blood transfusion Task Force. Br J Hematology.

TRANSFUSION IN STABLE ANAEMIC PATIENTS
Hgb <9 gm/dl
- Age > 65
- Known chr pulmonary disease or with symptoms of the same.
- Diabetes
- Cerebrovascular disease.
- PVD.

Hgb 7-9 gm/dl
Symptomatic patients with significant sustained compensatory mechanisms.

POTENTIAL ACUTE BLOOD LOSS OR SURGICAL STRESS IN STABLE ANAEMIC PATIENTS.
- Hgb <9-11 gm/dl : Known chr pulm or cerebrovascular disease and EBL of 1000 ml or 250 ml/hr.
- Hgb <7-9 gm/dl : All pts with EBL 1000ml or 250 ml/hr, surgical pts with hemostatic disorders or blood dyscrasias.
- Hgb <7 gm/dl : All patients in acute surgical stress.

CHOICE OF COMPONENT.

Leukoreduced red cell preparations:
- More costly
- Preferable in chronically transfused patients
- Potential transplant recipients
- Those with previous transfusion reactions
- CMV seronegative at risk in whom seronegative components are not available

Other Preparations:

Washed or Irradiated

Reinfusion of autologous red cells
Allow rapid transfusions of immense quantities.
Valuable for pts with antibodies.
May be acceptable to some Jehovah's witneses.
Damage cells to some degree.
Less than 10-15 L is recommended when possible.

MASSIVE BLOOD TRANSFUSIONS
Defined as the replacement of >50% of pts blood volume in 12- 24 hrs.
Each unit PRBCs has 300 ml volume, 200ml RBCs and will raise Hct by 3-4% in adults.
Oxygen release is diminished in transfused cells as they have reduced levels of 2,3-DPG. They regenerate this in 6-24hrs post transfusion.

COMPLICATIONS OF MASSIVE TRANSFUSION
ALTERATIONS IN COAGULATION SYSTEM –
- Patients may have pre-existing DIC or may develop it because of dilution.
- Approximately 10% decrease in the conc of clotting proteins for each 500 ml of blood loss that is replaced. Bleeding occurs at <25% of normal (i.e. 8-10 units of PRBC in adults.
- 2 units FFP if PT/PTT>1.5 times control. Each unit FFP will increase clotting proteins by 10%.
- Each 10-12 units of PRBCs can produce 50% fall in platelet count. 6 units platelets can be transfused in this setting. Each unit should increase count by 5000-10000.

METABOLIC ALKALOSIS
pH at time of collection is 7.1. It then falls by 0.1 per week, but acidosis does not develop as long as tissue perfusion is maintained.
Each mmol of Citrate generates 3meqs of HCO3 (for a total of 23 meqs HCO3 / unit PRBC).
Movement of K into cells.

HYPOCALCEMIA
secondary to citrate binding of ionized Ca.

HYPOTHERMIA
Commercial blood warmer recommended during massive blood transfusion.

HYPERKALEMIA
K increases by 1 meq/L/day due to passive leak. Na-K-ATPase inhibited at 1-6^C.
K conc peaks at 30 meq/L in whole blood & 90 meq/L in PRBC
Loss of 1unit of blood results in loss of 1.5 meq of K, which is replaced by 10 meqs in transfusion.
Significant in infants & those with renal impairment. In these blood collected <5 days prior to transfusion, whole blood packed immediately before infusion or PRBC washed immediately before infusion can be used.

RECOMMENDATIONS
- PT, aPTT & platelet count should be confirmed after every 5-7 units PRBCs. Replacement therapy should not be based on any formula.
- If platelet count falls below 50, 6 units platelets should be given.
- Maximum Citrate infusion (mmol/kg/min) = 1.33 * wt.(kg). This equals 8.9 units whole blood/hr or 33.3 units PRBCs/hr for a 50 kg recipient with normal hepatic function & perfusion.
- Plasma ionized Ca should be monitored in those with pre-existing liver disease or ischemia.
- 10-20 ml of 10% Ca-gluconate (or 2-5 ml Ca-chloride) in another vein for each 500ml blood.
- Blood warmer to be used when transfusing >3 units.
- Acid-Base balance, ionized Ca & K should be monitored in patients with liver & renal disease.

PLASMA PRODUCTS
FFP
Used within 24 hrs of thawingor the concentrations of Factors V & VIII begin to decline.
Needs to be ABO compatible but does not require Rh typing or cross-matching.

Indications -
- Emergency reversal of Warfarin
- Replacement of isola
- ted coag protein def.
- Massive transfusion & documented coag defect
- DIC
- Hypovolemic shock with coag defect unresponsive to platelets
- Liver disease with clinical coag defect
- TTP
- Severe protein losing enteropathy in infants

CRYOPRECIPITATE
Collected by thawing FFP at 4^C & collecting the white precipitate.
This is rich in vWF, factor VIII, XIII and Fibrinogen.
Much smaller obligate volume than FFP

Indications –
- Hemophilia A
- Von Willebrand Disease
- Fibrinogen def.
- Dysfibrinogenemia
- Factor XIII def.
- Uremic platelet dysfunction

LIQUID PLASMA
Prepared from previously stored whole blood
Low levels of factor V & VIII

FACTOR CONCENTRATES
Produced with Recombinant technology or collected from 1000s of donors & pooled into highly conc final product.
Indicated in specific factor deficiencies.
With minimal volume & no extraneous proteins.

DESMOPRESSIN (DDAVP)
Alternative to cryo-ppt or factor conc.
Causes release of Factor VIII:vWF multimers from endothelial cells